PHYTOTHERAPY
Fifty Vital Herbs

by Andrew Chevallier

BA (Hons) FNIMH

Published by
Amberwood Publishing Ltd
Guildford, England

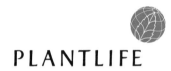

PLANTLIFE

The Natural History Museum, Cromwell Road, London SW7 5BD

Registered Charity No. 328576

Amberwood Publishing supports the Plantlife Charity,
Britain's only charity exclusively dedicated to saving wild plants.

ISBN 1-899308-19-9

Cover design by Howland Northover

Printed in Great Britain

CONTENTS

1.	Agnus Castus	9	26. Hawthorn	59
2.	Aloe Vera	11	27. Kava Kava	61
3.	Black Cohosh	13	28. Lemon Balm	63
4.	Buchu	15	29. Limeflower	65
5.	Burdock Root	16	30. Liquorice	67
6.	Capsicum Fruit	18	31. Lobelia	70
7.	Celery	20	32. Marigold	72
8.	Chamomile (German)	22	33. Milk Thistle	74
9.	Cornsilk	25	34. Nettle	76
10.	Cramp Bark	26	35. Parsley Piert	79
11.	Cranesbill (American)	28	36. Passiflora	80
12.	Damiana	30	37. Peppermint	82
13.	Dandelion Leaf	31	38. Raspberry	85
14.	Devil's Claw	34	39. Rosemary	87
15.	Echinacea	36	40. Sage	89
16.	Elderflower	38	41. Saw Palmetto	91
17.	Elecampane	40	42. St John's Wort	93
18.	Feverfew	42	43. Slippery Elm	96
19.	Garlic	44	44. Thyme	98
20.	Gentian	47	45. Valerian	100
21.	Ginger	49	46. Vervain	103
22.	Ginkgo	51	47. Wild Yam Root	105
23.	Ginseng: Chinese	53	48. Willow Bark	107
24.	Ginseng: Siberian	55	49. Witch Hazel	109
25.	Golden Seal	57	50. Wormwood	111

Note to Reader

About the Author

A practising medical herbalist, and Fellow and past President of the National Institute of Medical Herbalists, Andrew Chevallier is currently Senior Lecturer in Herbal Medicine at Middlesex University, having helped to pioneer and develop the 4-year BSc (Hons) course in Herbal Medicine there. He appears regularly on radio and television and is a leading figure in the world of complementary and alternative medicine. Other books by him include *Herbal First Aid* and *Natural Taste: Herbal Teas*, both published by Amberwood, and *The Encyclopedia of Medicinal Plants*.

Introduction

Fifty Vital Herbs may seem a strange title for a book on herbal medicine but perhaps the word *vital* conveys just how important these and similar herbs are to our health now and in the coming century. Not only are they as ecologically friendly as you can get, being a natural part of life on our planet, they are, by and large, equally friendly to the body's internal environment.

At a time when there is major concern over the ecological impact of antibiotics and synthesised chemical drugs, herbal medicine offers a chance to treat disease and encourage the return of good health in a way that is in accord with the needs of our environment – both internal and external. Moreover, clinical trials into herbs such as Ginger, Ginkgo, Peppermint and St John's Wort increasingly indicate that while their effect as medicines is directly comparable to conventional drugs, the herbal medicines have a very significantly lower incidence of side effects. Herbal medicines therefore, are not just useful substitutes for conventional medicines – they can be *better* medicines too.

This does not mean that herbal medicines are invariably safe or that *natural* medicines are always the appropriate ones to use, though it does mean that when used carefully and sensibly they can bring real therapeutic benefit.

All of the fifty herbs chosen form a key part of the canon of the western herbal tradition, having in many cases been used continuously as medicines for several thousands of years. Well-known and well-loved herbs like Elder, Rosemary, Sage and Yarrow have been used in medicine since long before Dioscorides published the first major European book on herbal medicine – *De Materia Medica* – in the 1st century AD. Other herbs such as Ginkgo are very recent arrivals in western herbal medicine, having been used in traditional Chinese medicine for thousands of years. And some herbs e.g. Garlic, have by now been so well researched that they are scientifically validated as medicines in their own right.

The information provided in each of the herb profiles gives a concise picture of the medicinal activity of the herb and how it may be used.

Sections on Habitat and Cultivation, and on Pharmacology/Research, have been kept deliberately short, and are pointers towards much more detailed knowledge to be found elsewhere. The same is true for Constituents, though I have tried to include all the known *active* constituents. The other sections can be used as a guide for the home use of herbal medicines, and as a good starting point for students of herbal medicine embarking on the study of *materia medica* (the term itself coming directly down through history from Dioscorides' work).

Dosages given are intended to reflect safe maximum levels for self-treatment, not necessarily the dosage used in professional practice. Relatively high doses can be used for short periods of time (generally up to one week) for acute conditions e.g. 'flu, tonsillitis; but much smaller doses are required for the long term treatment of chronic illness. Despite such information this book can *in no way* act as a substitute for the training and experience available from a medical herbalist or medical practitioner – if in doubt always seek professional herbal or medical advice.

Lastly, this introduction would be incomplete without reference to the other meaning of the title – *vital* in the sense of vitality.

From the time of Hippocrates (5th century BC) almost until the beginning of the 20th century, western medicine believed that robust health and resistance to illness was due to a *vital force* within the body, an organising and adaptive energy that enabled the living body to engage effectively with stresses and threats confronting it. Medical herbalists continue to use this idea when considering treatment, for herbs are as valuable in enhancing health and vitality – the capacity to meet and overcome challenge, as in treating disease.

The recent growth of psychoneuroimmunology, and of the awareness that emotional state and immune function are interlinked, suggest that the idea of a vital force, of an intimate connection between how we feel and our ability to act and adapt to the world, is not a convenient myth. Rather it is an accurate description of the powerful integrative and self-regenerating force that enables us to sustain ourselves when under extreme stress – physical, mental or emotional. Though not commonly acknowledged, herbal medicines work to support the body on this kind of level, supporting and strengthening our vital capacity to meet whatever challenges life throws at us – illness, bereavement, depression or simple exhaustion!

1 | *Vitex Agnus-Castus* – AGNUS CASTUS, CHASTE TREE
•••••••••••••••••••••••••••••••••••

Family: *Verbenaceae*

Habitat and cultivation
A native of the Mediterranean region and western Asia, Agnus Castus is cultivated in subtropical regions around the world, often becoming naturalised. The berries are collected when mature in the autumn, and dried.

CONSTITUENTS
Essential oil – (0.5-1.22%) including cineol and sabinene
Alkaloid – viticine
Flavonoids – casticin
Iridoids – aucubin, agnoside, eurostoside

Actions: Hormone regulator, progesterogenic, increases breast milk production.

Pharmacology/Research
Research into Agnus Castus has been going on for over 30 years. It has been established that the berries have a distinct hormonal effect on the body – increasing progesterone levels in women. They exert their action via the pituitary gland: increasing lutenising hormone and prolactin secretion, and decreasing follicle stimulating hormone secretion. Some clinical trials have shown Agnus Castus to be effective in pre-menstrual syndrome (PMS), and to increase fertility, though it is now suggested that Agnus Castus is effective in treating PMS only where a low progesterone level is associated with high prolactin levels. However, despite this research the constituents responsible for this hormonal activity have not been isolated. It is thought that Agnus Castus is best taken on waking in the morning when the hypothalamic-pituitary axis in the brain is most active. It is worthwhile following this suggestion and taking Agnus Castus once a day early in the morning.

Cautions: Excess doses can lead to infrequent menstruation. Do not take in combination with the contraceptive pill.

Parts used: Berries.

PREPARATIONS
Capsule – up to 1g each morning
Tincture (1:5) – up to 30ml per week

Key indications: Pre-menstrual syndrome especially breast tenderness, irregular periods, menopausal complaints, migraine linked to menstrual cycle, acne (in men and women).

Indications

An important hormonally-active herb, and to date the only herb with a progesterone-type activity, Agnus Castus is a key herb for menstrual problems, from pre-menstrual syndrome (PMS) and many of the symptoms that accompany it – such as breast swelling and tenderness, to irregular or absent periods. By increasing progesterogenic activity it appears to help balance progesterone and oestrogen production by the ovaries throughout the menstrual cycle. In PMS it should be taken for some months to see the full benefit, which can often be significant – with bloating, breast tenderness, irritability and depression all reduced. However it is unlikely to help and may make matters worse in symptoms in PMS type D (high progesterone, low oestrogen) which is characterised by depression, crying, confusion and insomnia. It is not particularly helpful for menstrual pains and cramps, though it will help to regulate irregular periods, tending to shorten a long cycle and lengthen a short cycle. Agnus Castus is valuable in treating migraines and acne when linked to the menstrual cycle, and can be valuable in severe cases of acne in men and women. In both cases, combined with appropriate herbs e.g. Feverfew or Echinacea, Agnus Castus can bring noticeable improvement. The berries increase breast milk production. Where infertility is due to low progesterone levels Agnus Castus can be very effective in aiding conception (always best to remember when taking Agnus Castus that it is likely to increase fertility).

COMBINATIONS
With Black Cohosh for pre-menstrual and menopausal problems
With Echinacea for acne with a hormonal cause
With Feverfew for menstrual migraine

2 | *Aloe Vera* – ALOE VERA
•••••••••••••••••••••••

Family: *Liliaceae*

Habitat and cultivation
Aloe Vera is native to eastern and southern Africa, but is now found in tropical regions across the world. It is cultivated extensively. The leaves are cut and the clear sap collected. Plants grown to produce aloe vera gel have been selected for their low anthraquinone content.

CONSTITUENTS
Anthraquinone glycosides – aloin, aloe-emodin
Resins; Tannins
Polysaccharides
Aloectin B

Key actions: Emollient to skin, wound and tissue healer.

Pharmacology/Research
The anthraquinones, present in the dried yellow sap (= 'bitter Aloes') produce an irritant laxative effect similar to Senna. Plants grown for the gel have only a very mild laxative activity. The clear sap i.e. the gel, derived from the leaves is a very effective would healer, in part due to Aloectin B which is an immunostimulant, which also stimulates tissue repair. Extensive research across the world, and particularly in the USA and Russia since the 1940s, has confirmed Aloe Vera's remarkable ability to heal wounds, burns and inflammatory skin conditions. Most famously studies have shown that Aloe Vera gel aids the healing of radiation burns.

11

Other species: *A. ferox* (Cape Aloes) native to Southern Africa is a close relative used as a laxative. Many other species of Aloe are also useful medicinally, mainly as laxatives.

Cautions: Do not take internally during pregnancy or while breast-feeding. Avoid in kidney disease, and be cautious if haemorrhoids are present.

Parts used: Clear gel; dried yellow sap.

PREPARATIONS
Gel – 'grow your own' and press the clear gel from fresh leaf or purchase commercially clarified gel.

Key indications: Externally: wound, burn and scar healing; many skin disorders e.g. acne; varicose veins and ulcers. Internally: Gastritis, peptic ulcers, irritable bowel, inflammatory bowel problems such as ulcerative colitis.

Indications
Despite Aloe Vera's reputation as a lotion for the skin – Cleopatra is said to have attributed her beauty to Aloe gel – it is only since its ability to heal burns, and in particular radiation burns, was 'discovered' in the 50s that it has become popular in the west. It has a dramatic ability to heal wounds, burns and other skin problems, putting a protective coat on the affected area, and speeding the rate of healing. Like Comfrey its tissue regenerating activity makes it potentially useful in healing scars and keloid tissue. Being easily grown indoors it makes an excellent first aid treatment in domestic accidents, the sap being released as soon as a leaf is broken. It is useful in almost any skin condition which needs soothing and astringing, and can help varicose veins. Internally, the gel can be used for peptic ulcers, its protective and regenerative effect working topically within the gut. Recently it has become popular in the treatment of irritable bowel. In view of its immuno-modulating activity it can be valuable in other gut related illness e.g. ulcerative colitis, rheumatoid arthritis, etc. Aloes, or bitter Aloes, is used as a bitter tonic at low doses, stimulating the digestion in general, and as a laxative and purgative at higher doses.

COMBINATIONS
Topically – with Marigold/Calendula for inflamed skin
Internally – with Geranium and Peppermint for irritable bowel syndrome

3 | *Cimicifuga Racemosa* – BLACK COHOSH

Family: *Ranunculaceac*

Habitat and cultivation
Native to eastern USA and Canada, preferring mainly shaded positions in woods and hedgerows. It is cultivated in Europe and can sometimes be found as a garden escape. The rootstock is harvested and dried after the aerial parts have died down in the autumn.

CONSTITUENTS
Triterpene glycosides – actein, cimicifugoside
Isoflavones – formononetin
Isoferulic acid
Salicylic acid
Tannins
Rein

Key actions: Emmenagogue, antirheumatic, expectorant, sedative.

Pharmacology/Research
Black Cohosh has an established oestrogenic activity, in part due to isoflavones including formononetin. It reduces pituitary luteinizing hormone (LH) levels – LH increases progesterone production by the ovaries. It is thought that the triterpenes have a direct effect on the pituitary gland and hypothalamus within the brain. A number of clinical

trials (mostly in Germany) have indicated Black Cohosh's value in menopausal problems, especially aiding in reducing hot flushing. One recent trial reported at the 1995 International Conference of Phytotherapy in Berlin showed improvements in symptoms such as menopausal hot flushing of up to 90% (this trial combined Black Cohosh with St John's Wort).

Other species
Other Cohosh's are used in Chinese herbal medicine, including *C. foetida* and *C. dahurica*. These are used for asthma, measles and headaches and other conditions.

Cautions: Do not take during pregnancy or while breastfeeding.

Parts used: Root.

PREPARATIONS
Capsule – up to 1g daily
Tincture (1:5) – up to 35ml per week

Key indications: Cramps, sciatic pains; painful periods and pre-menstrual tension; menopausal hot flushing; tinnitus; rheumatic disorders.

Indications
Native American Indians used this plant for menstrual and menopausal problems, and as one of its traditional names Squaw Root implies it is first and foremost a woman's herb. It is used most often today to relieve menstrual cramps and pains, menstrual problems where oestrogen production is too low, and particularly for menopausal problems including hot flushing, debility and depression, where it can be *extremely* helpful. Black Cohosh is equally useful for rheumatic problems including rheumatoid arthritis and for inflammatory arthritis, especially when associated with the menopause. Useful also for headaches. It is a herb to think of in cases of osteoporosis. Its sedative activity makes it of value in high blood pressure and tinnitus (combine with Ginkgo), and whooping cough and asthma. The Chinese Cimicifuga's are thought to clear heat, relieve toxicity and are used to treat 'wind-heat' patterns of illness.

COMBINATIONS
With Wild Yam for menopausal problems and for inflammatory arthritis
e.g. rheumatoid arthritis
With St John's Wort for hot flushing
With Ginkgo for tinnitus

4 | *Barosma Betulina* – BUCHU
•••••••••••••••••••••••••

Family: *Rutaceae*

Habitat and cultivation
Native to South Africa and also grown in parts of South America. Widely cultivated in South Africa preferring sunny hillsides. It is collected when in flower and fruiting.

CONSTITUENTS
Volatile oil (1.5-2.5%) – pulegone, menthone, diosphenol
Sulphur compounds
Flavonoids – diosmin, rutin
Mucilage

Actions: Urinary antiseptic, diuretic, stimulant.

Pharmacology/Research
Very little research exists on Buchu. Diosphenol is diuretic, and may be partly responsible for the observed antiseptic action.

Cautions: Avoid in pregnancy.

Parts used: Leaves.

PREPARATIONS
Infusion/Douche – up to 2g three times a day
Capsule – up to 1g a day
Tincture (1:5) – up to 40ml per week

Key indications: Cystitis, urethritis, flatulence.

Indications
Buchu is a traditional southern African remedy used as a stimulant and diuretic, and being strongly aromatic as a carminative – helping to relieve wind and bloating. It was first exported to Britain in 1790 and became an official medicine in 1821, being listed 'as a remedy for cystitis, urethritis, nephritis and catarrh of the bladder'. Broadly speaking this is its current use in herbal medicine though it finds use in prostatitis and irritable bladder as well. It is generally used mixed with other herbs. For cystitis, take as an infusion or tincture – the infusion being preferable for cystitis with a sudden onset. Buchu may be used as a douche in leucorrhea, and occasionally for thrush. It has a distinct aroma of blackcurrants.

COMBINATIONS
With Damiana for cystitis
With Willow bark for prostatitis

5 | *Arctium Lappa* – BURDOCK ROOT
•••••••••••••••••••••••••••••••••

Family: *Compositae*

Habitat and cultivation
Native to Europe and Asia and found throughout temperate regions, Burdock thrives in meadows, glades and as a wayside plant. Cultivated in Europe and China. The plant is dug up in July and the root and leaves dried; the seeds are picked when ripe.

CONSTITUENTS
Root: Bitter glycosides – arctiopicrin
Flavonoids – arctiin
Alkaloid; Tannins; Polyacetylenes; Volatile oil; Inulin (up to 45%)

Key actions: Detoxicant, mild diuretic, antibiotic, mild bitter.

Pharmacology/Research
The polyacetylenes are antibiotic, especially in the fresh root; arctiin is a smooth muscle relaxant. The plant has been shown to have antibacterial and antifungal properties (seed), and diuretic and hypoglycaemic effects. Burdock appears to have an anti-tumour activity.

Cautions: Use with care when treating conditions resulting from poor elimination or significant toxicity, as more than small doses may precipitate a short term 'flare up' in symptoms e.g. eczema. Avoid during pregnancy and breastfeeding.

Parts used: Leaf, root, fruit (seeds).

PREPARATIONS
Decoction (root) – up to 5g a day; almost invariably in combination with other herbs
Juice (leaf/stem) – traditionally used for baldness (topical application)
Capsule – up to 1g a day
Tincture (1:5) – up to 40ml per week

Key indications: Skin disorders such as acne, boils, atopic and sebhorrheic eczema, skin infections in general; fevers, and acute infections of the throat, e.g. tonsillitis, quinsy; chronic infections of all kinds; detoxification, e.g. lead poisoning, mercury poisoning from tooth fillings.

Indications
Classically used in both western and Chinese traditions to aid detoxification in fevers and infections such as tonsillitis, mumps and measles (combine with Echinacea and Phytolacca), Burdock supports

elimination in acute *and* chronic skin conditions, as well as in arthritis (mainly the root). With diuretic, antibiotic and mildly bitter activity Burdock has a place in prescriptions for skin disorders of all kinds, especially where toxicity is a key factor – acne, boils, abscesses and local skin infections – and is often used in eczema and psoriasis. Rarely used on its own it is combined with other herbs to balance its strong eliminative activity. It is thought to draw toxins out of the cells into the interstitial fluid, and thence in to the blood. As a result if given in too high a dosage it will lead to a rapid increase in toxins/metabolites within the blood leading to aggravation of skin problems. As a rule start with a low dosage, and slowly increase. May be used where heavy metal toxicity is suspected – Burdock is thought to specifically aid elimination of heavy metals such as lead. It is one of the herbs in formulations commonly taken to aid detoxification in cancer.

COMBINATIONS
With Dandelion as the standard combination for skin problems such as acne and boils. Also with Echinacea and Marigold
With Marigold and Echinacea for chronic infections e.g. tonsillitis, lymphadenopathy
With Echinacea, Thyme and Golden Seal for candidiasis

6 | *Capsicum Frutescens* – CAPSICUM FRUIT

Family: *Solanaceae*

Habitat
Native to the tropical Americas, and grown throughout the tropics, especially Africa and India.

CONSTITUENTS
Capsaicin (0.1-1.5%)
Carotenoids
Flavonoids
Volatile oil
Steroidal saponins (seeds and root only) – capsicidin

Key actions: Stimulant, tonic, carminative, spasmolytic, antiseptic, diaphoretic, counterirritant.

Pharmacology/Research
Capsaicin produces a wide range of effects on the body including stimulating the circulation and altering temperature regulation of the body, where it lowers the body temperature setting. Capsicum as a whole however is used to support those liable to cold and hypothermia. It is thought to stimulate metabolic rate by up to 25%. It may be used as a local analgesic as its acrid effect on sensory nerves leads to desensitisation, and the stimulation of endorphin release. Capsicidin has antibiotic properties.

Cautions: Avoid in cases of peptic ulcer, acid digestion and skin rashes e.g. eczema.

Parts used: Fruit – fresh or dried.

PREPARATIONS
Tincture; capsules and tablets.

Key indications: Poor peripheral circulation; chilblains; weak digestion; hypothermia; low metabolic rate. Topically on cold extremities or joints.

Indications
Capsicum's heating qualities make it specific for 'cold' conditions, typically poor peripheral circulation – good therefore for chilblains, and in all situations requiring circulatory stimulation e.g. bronchitis. It may be added to many prescriptions as an adjuvant, adding force to the prescription, being thought to improve the distribution of the medicine

as a whole through the body. Internally, Cayenne makes an excellent addition to gargles – add a pinch to honey, lemon and hot water. It relieves wind and colic, and stimulates the secretion of digestive juices. Is antiseptic within the digestive system, will counter infection if present, and can be a useful medicine in some cases of dysentery and diarrhoea. It raises stomach acid production and therefore helps prevent digestive infection. May be used for chronic fatigue and to raise body temperature. Use often in winter! Applied locally to the skin it is mildly analgesic and irritant. This 'counter- irritant' effect is employed to stimulate the circulation in 'cold' rheumatic and arthritic problems – aiding the removal of waste products and increasing nutrition to the area. Cayenne is also used as a paint on unbroken chillblains. For those prone to permanently cold feet – a traditional remedy involves putting Cayenne powder in one's socks. Add drops of Chilli sauce to their food or take capsules regularly throughout the winter.

COMBINATIONS
With Celery and Willow Bark for osteoarthritis
With Cranesbill for diarrhoea

7 | *Apium Graveolens* – CELERY

Family: *Umbelliferae*

Habitat and cultivation
A marshland plant that grows best in damp places Celery is native to Britain amongst other countries, and is often found along the English and Welsh coasts. Grown throughout temperate regions of the world as a vegetable, the cultivated variety is less fragrant than in its wild state. The plant is harvested from June to October.

CONSTITUENTS
Volatile oil (1.5-3%) – limonene (60-70%), B-selinene
Coumarins
Furanocoumarins – bergapten
Flavonoids – apiin

Key actions: Diuretic, urinary antiseptic, anti-rheumatic, anti-spasmodic, hypotensive.

Pharmacology/Research
The volatile oil has been shown to have a tranquillising effect on the central nervous system, with some of its constituents having anti-spasmodic, sedative, anti-convulsant and sedative activity. Studies in China have confirmed its usefulness in high blood pressure.

Cautions: Avoid in kidney disorders and pregnancy.

Parts used: Fruit (seeds).

PREPARATIONS
Cooking – vegetable and seeds
Juice of stems – cleansing and detoxifying
Crushed/powdered seeds – sprinkle ½ tsp on food a day
Capsules – up to 1.5g a day
Tincture (1:5) – up to 50ml per week

Key indications: Rheumatic and arthritic disorders including osteoarthritis, gout and rheumatoid arthritis; cystitis; high blood pressure; flatulence; to increase breast milk production.

Indications
Celery has been cultivated for at least 3,000 years, notably in pharaonic Egypt, and was known in China in the 5th century BC. At different times the plant as a whole or the seeds have been used as a medicine, though the plant has been used as food throughout this time. The seeds are more or less a specific in rheumatic conditions and gout, supporting kidney clearance of urates and other unwanted waste products, and reducing

acidity in the body as a whole. Celery appears to have some anti-inflammatory activity and will often prove useful in 'hot' arthritic conditions including osteoarthritis. It may also be used for 'cold' conditions, stimulating detoxification via the kidneys and improved circulation to muscles and joints. The seeds are diuretic, and disinfect the bladder and urinary tubules – a decoction of the seeds (and the juice of the plant) makes an effective treatment for mild cystitis. The seeds may be given in chest problems such as asthma and bronchitis, and (in combination with e.g. Hawthorn) aid in lowering the blood pressure. Celery and carrot juices combined are highly nutritious and cleansing suitable for almost all chronic illness.

COMBINATIONS
With Willow Bark for gout and arthritis
With Buchu for cystitis

8 | *Chamomilla Recutita* – GERMAN CHAMOMILE
●●●●●●●●●●●●●●●●●●●●●●●●

Family: *Compositae*

Habitat and cultivation
Grows wild and cultivated in much of Europe but now grown in many countries including Egypt, North America and Argentina. It prefers previously cultivated soils. The fresh flowerheads are picked when in full bloom generally from May to August. Dry in shade below 35°C. NB. max. content of active constituents is several days after blooming.

CONSTITUENTS
Volatile oil – proazulenes, bisabolol, farnesine, spiroether
Flavonoids – anthemedin, luteolin, rutin
Bitter glycosides – anthemic acid
Coumarins; Malic acid; Tannins

Actions: Anti-inflammatory, antispasmodic, relaxant, carminative, mild bitter, anti-catarrhal.

Pharmacology/Research
The volatile oil contains strongly anti-inflammatory and anti- spasmodic compounds – the proazulenes – which on steam distillation produce chamazulene. This compound is markedly anti-allergenic, and indicates that Chamomile may also be used for allergic and spasmodic states such as asthma and hay fever. Spiroether in isolation is a stronger antispasmodic than papaverine – found in the opium poppy, and the herb as a whole has clearly established anti-inflammatory and antispasmodic effects. German research has established Chamomile as an effective wound healer and local anti-inflammatory, making it a good remedy for red and inflamed skin problems.

Other species
Though German Chamomile and *Chamaemelum nobile* (Roman Chamomile) are used interchangeably there is a significant difference in their constituents, notably the volatile oil which in Chamaemelum has no chamazulene.

Cautions: No side effects are known but allergic reactions occur occasionally.

Parts used: Flowerheads.

PREPARATIONS
Infusion – up to 15g a day; always prepare infusion in a closed container
Capsules – up to 3g a day
Tincture (1:5) – up to 60ml per week
Lotion – use infusion
Essential oil – dilute to 5% for topical use; for short term can be sniffed for hay fever
Cream – for sore and tender skin
Bath – use 25-50g to a litre of water
Teabag – good compress for sore inflamed eyes

Key indications: Fractiousness, irritability and teething in children; insomnia and restlessness; nervous and muscular tension; digestive cramps and discomfort; acidic indigestion; pre-menstrual tension and period cramps; catarrhal states.

Indications

Chamomile is specific for gastritis, hiatus hernia, peptic ulceration, and almost any digestive problem linked to nervous tension. Dioscorides (1st century AD) states that 'it is an excellent and very familiar remedy against an infinite number of infirmities that afflict the human body'. It finds a place in many prescriptions. Frequently prescribed for upper abdominal pain, cramps, indigestion, acidity, wind, bloating: and for colic, regional ileitis (Crohn's disease), ulcerative colitis and irritable bowel syndrome. Use also for nervous tension, muscle pain and period cramps. For over-excitability, irritability, fractiousness and sleep disturbance, especially in young children. The strained infusion can be added to a bath when the child will not drink it. Chamomile's anti-allergenic and antispasmodic activity makes it of use in hay fever and asthma – as a steam inhalation, tincture or infusion. Apply as a lotion, ointment or cream on sores, sore nipples/mastitis, leg ulcers, itchiness and eczema. A warm teabag or flowerheads placed on closed eyes is very soothing and relieves tired and strained eyes.

COMBINATIONS

For gastrointestinal problems associated with nervous interference and anxiety – with Valerian

For flatulent dyspepsia – with Peppermint and Sage

For all inflammatory states within the upper digestive tract e.g. peptic ulcer – with Cranesbill

24

9 | *Zea Mays* – CORNSILK, MAIZE

Family: *Graminae*

Habitat and cultivation

A well known and almost universally cultivated food crop, Corn is native to the Andes and central America, possibly originating in Peru. Cornsilk is harvested with the corn cob when ripe, separated and dried.

CONSTITUENTS

Flavonoids – maysin
Alkaloid; allantoin; volatile oil – about 0.2%
Mucilage; saponins; potassium

Actions: Urinary demulcent, diuretic, mild cholagogue, mild hypotensive.

Pharmacology/Research

Cornsilk has an established diuretic action, increasing urine production partly due to the significant level of potassium present. The mucilage is thought to contribute to the herbs soothing activity within the kidneys and urinary tract. It is also thought to be cholagogic improving the bile flow through the bile ducts. Allantoin is a potent tissue healer. Research in China indicates that Cornsilk tends to reduce blood pressure and blood clotting time.

Cautions: For kidney problems use under professional guidance only.

Parts used: Stigma (the silken fronds) – fresh or dried; meal – for external use.

PREPARATIONS

Infusion (stigma) – up to 25g a day
Capsules (stigma) – up to 5g a day
Decoction (meal) – can be used as a lotion or poultice for sores, boils, etc.
Tincture (stigma))(1:5) 25% – up to 15ml a day

Indications

Cornsilk may be prescribed for almost any problem affecting the urinary system. It has a beneficial action on the kidneys, traditionally being considered to reduce kidney stone formation and to relieve some of the symptoms of existing kidney stones. As a demulcent it appears to have a soothing and relaxing action on the lining of the urinary tubules and bladder, relieving irritation and improving urine flow and elimination. Use for chronic cystitis, general irritation to the bladder and urethral walls, and in situations where passing urine is difficult e.g. prostate enlargement. In acute cystitis Cornsilk is a useful adjunct to other treatment, where it is often best taken as an infusion. Cornmeal makes an effective poultice and has been used in Mayan, Incan and American folk medicine to treat bruises, swellings, sores and boils. Early Europeans arriving in the Americas noted with amazement that native Americans rarely if ever suffered from kidney or bladder problems, and put it down to the fact that Corn was the staple food in their diet.

COMBINATIONS
With Echinacea and Buchu for acute and chronic cystitis
With Parsley Piert for kidney stones

10 | *Viburnum Opulus* – CRAMP BARK
●●●●●●●●●●●●●●●●●●●●●●●●●●●●●●●●

Family: *Caprifoliaceae*

Habitat and cultivation

Cramp Bark is found in damp woods, hedges and thickets through much of Europe and eastern North America. The branch bark is collected in spring and summer, when the plant is in flower.

CONSTITUENTS
Hydroquinones – arbutin; Coumarins – scopoletin; Tannins – 3%; Resin

Key actions: Antispasmodic, sedative, astringent, nervine

Pharmacology/Research
A poorly researched herb with some confusion over what active constituents occur within Cramp Bark (*Viburnum opulus*) as opposed Black Haw Bark (*V. prunifolium*).

Other species: Black Haw Bark is a very close relative often used interchangeably with Cramp Bark, though the former possibly has a more specific action on the womb.

Cautions: None.

Parts used: Bark.

PREPARATIONS
Infusion – up to 15g a day for short term use e.g. period pains
Capsules – up to 3g a day
Tincture (1:5) 45% – up to 20ml a day

Key indications: Muscle cramps associated with arthritis, sprains and back pain; nervous tension; menstrual cramps; colic and irritable bowel; asthma; high blood pressure.

Indications
Perhaps the most useful spamolytic of all, Cramp Bark may be used in any situation where muscle tension – whether visceral or skeletal – is a key factor. In both cases Cramp Bark will reduce muscle tension and spasticity relieving pain and improving blood flow to the affected area. Possible uses for the herb are therefore wide ranging and include: high blood pressure, osteoarthritis, asthma and bronchitis, angina and intermittent claudication, menstrual cramps, spastic constipation, irritable bladder and bowel, nervous tension, and the symptomatic reduction in muscle spasticity due to cerebral palsy. Cramp Bark can occasionally bring dramatic relief to chronic back pain – as muscles relax so blood flow to the area improves, waste products such as lactic acid are removed, and normal movement and function can begin to return. It is usually best used in combination with herbs that have a specific activity on the area needing attention.

COMBINATIONS
With Valerian and Chamomile for colic and irritable bowel
With St John's Wort for spasmodic back pain
With Lobelia (topical use) as a general purpose anti-spasmodic lotion
With Valerian and Hawthorn for high blood pressure
With Lobelia, Ginkgo and Liquorice in asthma

11 | *Geranium Maculatum* – AMERICAN CRANESBILL
••••••••••••••••••••••••••

Family: *Geraniaceae*

Habitat and cultivation
Found commonly in woodlands over most of eastern and central North America, Cranesbill root is gathered before the plant flowers in late winter and early spring, the herb when in flower in spring.

CONSTITUENTS
Tannins – up to 30%

Actions: Astringent

Pharmacology/Research
As with all remedies containing appreciable quantities of tannins, one can be certain that Cranesbill has a strongly astringent action – tightening up tissue with which it comes into contact. The root has a higher tannin content than the herb. Cranesbill has not been researched.

Cautions: Take internally for no more than 3-4 weeks at a time.

Parts used: Root, herb.

PREPARATIONS
Capsule – up to 600mg a day

Key indications: Internal bleeding e.g. from peptic ulcer, dysentery, diarrhoea; topically – haemorrhoids, ulcers, weeping skin conditions; sore throats – as a gargle.

Indications

An effective astringent and haemostatic, American Cranesbill still finds use for many of the disorders for which it was traditionally used by native Americans – for internal bleeding including the vomiting of blood, blood in the stool, or in the urine, diarrhoea, dysentery, and problems affecting the mucus membranes of the mouth and throat. It is commonly prescribed by herbalists for conditions such as irritable bowel and haemorrhoids. As a good haemostatic American Cranesbill is useful for wounds, slowing or stopping bleeding and encouraging regeneration and healing. It may be used for excessive menstrual bleeding and as a douche for leucorrhea (vaginal discharge). As with all herbs with a high tannin content it should not be taken for more than a few weeks at a time, as the astringent action of the tannins reduces the ability of the gut to successfully absorb nutrients. As might be expected of an astringent herb, American Cranesbill may be used as a gargle and mouthwash for pharyngitis, mouth ulcers, soggy and infected gums, and oral thrush. The Meskawi Indians used 'an infusion of the root for sore gums and pyorrhoea, toothache, neuralgia, piles and haemorrhoids' (Vogel, *American Indian Medicine* 1970). It was esteemed by American settlers, and used regularly to treat diarrhoea, dysentery, cholera and venereal diseases.

COMBINATIONS
With Chamomile for diarrhoea and irritable bowel

12 | *Turnera Diffusa* – DAMIANA

Family: *Turneraceae*

Habitat and cultivation
Native to the Gulf of Mexico, southern California and the northern Caribbean islands Damiana grows wild and in cultivation in the region, preferring a hot, humid climate.

CONSTITUENTS
Arbutin up to 7%
Volatile oil about 0.5% – D-cadinene (10%), thymol (4%)
Cyanogenic glycoside – tetraphyllin
Resins
Gums

Actions: Anti-depressant, tonic, stimulant, mild laxative, mild diuretic, reputed aphrodisiac.

Pharmacology/Research
An American herb which has had next to no detailed research undertaken into it. Arbutin, found in a number of other plant species notably Bearberry (*Arctostaphylos uva-ursi*) is converted in the urinary tubules in to hydroquinone a strong urinary antiseptic. Thymol is antiseptic and tonic. What little research there has been has been inconclusive, but as Potter's Cyclopaedia of Botanical Drugs and Preparations delicately puts it: 'The aphrodisiac activity has not yet been demonstrated experimentally, however this is very difficult to do'!

Parts used: Leaves – make a pleasant tasting tea.

PREPARATIONS
Infusion – up to 5g a day
Capsule – up to 2g a day
Tincture – up to 50ml per week

Key indications: Impotence, frigidity, prostatitis, nervous tiredness, mild depression and physical weakness.

Indications
Damiana is an excellent tonic and restorative for the nervous system and has always been considered an aphrodisiac. Technically, it is a thymoleptic (having a life enhancing and stimulating action on the body and mind), and is given in cases of mild to moderate depression and nervous exhaustion. Its combination of stimulation and restoration makes it a valuable remedy where anxiety and depression occur together, as is so often the case after long term stress. It has always been seen principally as a 'male' herb, helpful in treating impotence and premature ejaculation, though it is beneficial for both men and women, being considered restorative to the reproductive organs of both sexes. Damiana is also given for painful and delayed periods, and is used as a specific for menstrual headaches. Being mildly laxative and diuretic and a urinary antiseptic, it is useful in atonic constipation and urinary infections such as cystitis and urethritis. A Mayan herb, Damiana has always been used traditionally as an aphrodisiac. Its leaves are used in Mexico as a substitute for 'ordinary' Tea (*Camellia sinensis*), and to flavour liqueurs. It has a strongly aromatic and slightly bitter taste.

COMBINATIONS
With St John's Wort for depression
With Vitex and Feverfew for menstrual migraine

13 | *Taraxacum Officinale* – DANDELION LEAF

Family: *Compositae*

Habitat and cultivation
Dandelion grows throughout most of the world and is cultivated in many

countries, notably Germany and France. It grows in sunny sites in pastures, meadows and waysides. The leaves are picked early in the year as a vegetable, later as a medicine. The roots of two year old plants are unearthed in the autumn.

CONSTITUENTS
Sesquiterpene lactones
Triterpenes
Coumarins
Carotenoids
Vitamins A,B,C,D
Minerals, especially potassium

Actions: Diuretic, bitter, cholagogue/choleretic.

Pharmacology/Research
Dandelion leaf and root have been fairly well researched. The leaf (and to a lesser extent the root) has an established diuretic action, comparable in strength to orthodox diuretics such as frusemide, though large quantities must be taken to exert an equivalent effect. The leaf's mode of action in stimulating urine output by the kidneys and its flow through the urinary tubules is not understood. Unlike conventional diuretics which lead to a net loss of potassium, Dandelion contains such high levels of potassium, that there is thought to be a net gain of this mineral. Both leaf and root are cholagogues and stimulate the production and flow of bile from the liver through the bile ducts. They are thought to exert a significant detoxifying action on the liver, the root being considered more effective than the leaf in this area. The sesquiterpene lactones are appreciably bitter and stimulate appetite and digestive activity. The leaves are rich in vitamins and minerals and make a good salad vegetable and nutrient.

Cautions: A very safe herb – to be avoided only in severe pathology affecting the kidneys or gall-bladder/bile ducts.

Parts used: Leaves; roots.

PREPARATIONS
Leaves – in salads
Infusion, (leaf) – up to 7g a day
Capsule – up to 3g a day
Tincture (1:5) – up to 100ml per week

Key indications: Water retention; abdominal bloating; high blood pressure; sluggish gall bladder; gallstones.

Indications
Dandelion has a central place in herbal medicine being one of the most commonly used detoxifying herbs. Working principally on the liver and gallbladder, and on the kidneys, it stimulates the removal of waste via the bile and in the urine. Given the high level of pollutants our bodies are exposed to Dandelion root and leaf represent remarkably well-balanced remedies, encouraging the steady elimination of toxins resulting from infection or environmental pollution – the leaf having its main activity on the kidneys, the root on the liver. Both leaf and root can be of value in arthritic conditions such as osteoarthritis and gout, and being a powerful diuretic Dandelion leaf may be prescribed for any condition where fluid retention is a problem e.g. swollen ankles or bloated abdomen, and premenstrual fluid retention. As a diuretic it may be used by herbalists in the treatment of high blood pressure, reducing the overall fluid volume in the body. Both leaf and root also have a marked action on the gall bladder and are used to prevent gallstone formation. The leaf may possibly also help to dissolve already formed gallstones.

COMBINATIONS
With Celery seed and Willow Bark for gout and osteoarthritis
With Hawthorn and Garlic for high blood pressure

14 | *Harpagophytum Procumbens* – DEVIL'S CLAW
●●●●●●●●●●●●●●●

Family: *Pedaliaceae*

Habitat and cultivation
A native of southern and eastern Africa, particularly in the desert steppes of the Transvaal, Devil's Claw thrives in clayey, sandy soil. The young secondary side roots are unearthed in autumn, cut into approx. 2cm pieces and dried quickly to prevent mould growth.

CONSTITUENTS
Iridoid glycosides (0.5-3.0%) – mainly harpagoside, also harpagide and procumbide
Phenolic glycosides
Sugars – stachyose
Phytosterols – mainly B-sitosterol
Triterpenes
Flavonoids
Harpagoquinone

Actions: Anti-inflammatory, analgesic, anti-rheumatic, digestive stimulant, anti-arrythmic, hypotensive.

Pharmacology/Research
Devil's Claw appears to have an anti-inflammatory effect, however opinion is divided on its effectiveness in practice. It is likely that it has most effect (iridoid glycosides) in subacute inflammatory arthritic conditions, and clinical trials – see ESCOP monograph – tend to bear this out, as they do the herb's use for relieving back pain. It is strongly bitter (harpagoside), stimulating and toning up the digestive system. Devil's Claw is also hypotensive and decreases heart rate. The active constituents occur only in the storage roots, adulteration with the main root can render the remedy ineffective. Devil's Claw is best taken in enteric-coated form as stomach acidity reduces its therapeutic efficacy.

Cautions: Avoid in cases of stomach or duodenal ulcer. Best avoided during pregnancy.

Parts used: Secondary tubers.

PREPARATIONS
Capsule – up to 2g a day

Key indications: Osteoarthritis, rheumatoid arthritis, other arthropathies, digestive weakness, indigestion and flatulence, fever.

Indications
Used by various peoples in southern Africa, including the Bantu's, Devil's Claw is traditionally used as a tonic especially for digestive problems, for arthritis and rheumatism, to reduce fevers, and as an ointment applied to sores, ulcers and boils. Current western use draws significantly on these traditional therapeutic applications and the root is commonly prescribed for arthritic and rheumatic conditions such as gout, osteoarthritis, fibrositis and rheumatoid arthritis. Its analgesic action makes it of value where pain is a significant feature (often in combination with Willow Bark) but it will also tend to reduce associated inflammation and oedema. It may need to be used for some weeks for best results. Arthritic conditions are often associated with poor digestive function so that its stimulant activity on the stomach and gall bladder contributes to its overall therapeutic value as an anti-arthritic. It finds a place in many prescriptions for joint problems.

COMBINATIONS
With Black Cohosh and St John's Wort for rheumatoid arthritis
With Willow Bark for osteoarthritis

15 | *Echinacea Angustifolia and Purpurea* – PURPLE CONEFLOWER
•••••••••••••••••••••••••

Family: *Compositae*

Habitat and cultivation
Native to the central and southwestern United States, especially the Prairies, Echinacea is now cultivated extensively as a medicinal plant – from seed or divided crown – in USA and Europe (mainly *purpurea*), Echinacea likes sandy, fertile soils, and may take a lot of manuring. The roots should be planted out in the winter months in a sunny position. Protect from slugs.

CONSTITUENTS
Alkamides – highest in *E. angustifolia radix* (0. 15%)
– mostly isobutylamides with olefinic and acetylenic bonds; echinacein
Caffeic acid esters – highest in *E. purpurea flos and rad* – mainly echinacoside, and cichoric acid
Polysaccharides
Polyacetylenes
Volatile oil – highest in *E. pallida* (4% in May) – including humulene
Echinolone
Betaine
Pyrollizidine alkaloids – tussilagin (0.006%) and isotussilagin.

Actions: Immune stimulant, anti–inflammatory, anti–bacterial, anti–viral, anti–fungal, alterative, warming, diaphoretic, vulnerary, anti–allergenic.

Pharmacology/Research
Though extensively researched Echinacea's ability to stimulate the immune system is not yet fully understood. The polysaccharides inhibit the ability of viruses to enter and take over cells within the body (anti-hyaluronidase activity). The polyacetylenes are immune stimulant (as in the roots of other Compositae e.g. Burdock). At the same time the alkamides are anti bacterial and anti–fungal. Echinacein is responsible for

the plant's slightly pungent and anaesthetic action on the tongue. Besides these direct antipathogen effect, Echinacea appears to stimulate the body's non-specific immune defences to counter infection in general, increasing interleukin production, tumour necrosis factor and interferons. It also increases antibody production. The pyrollizidine alkaloids are not hepatotoxic. For further details see *Indian Medicine – The Immune System* by Corrigan. D (1994) Amberwood.

Other species: E. *pallida* is also used medicinally.

Cautions: No known side effects.

Parts used: Root and Rhizome.

PREPARATIONS
Decoction – up 5g a day
Capsule – maximum of 2.5g a day
Tincture (1:5) – up to 80ml a week (short-term use only at this level)

Key indications: Upper respiratory tract infection – acute, chronic and as a prophylactic; other chronic infections including chronic fatigue syndrome; acne, boils and other skin infections; allergic problems.

Indications
Echinacea is the most important immune stimulant in western herbal medicine. It can be used to treat infections of all kinds, and is particularly effective in chronic infections e.g. chronic fatigue syndrome (ME), in skin infections such as acne and boils, and wherever there is underlying toxicity within the body. It is probably most often of use however, as a preventative, helping to reduce the likelihood of developing colds, flu and other upper respiratory tract infections. Recent developments in immunology suggest that the immune system and the emotions are closely connected, and Echinacea's ability to warm and to raise vitality parallels its ability to stimulate immune function. Echinacea is probably most useful for throat problems such as tonsillitis and quinsy, where it can also be used as a gargle, and the whole plant has been shown to help in

the treatment of allergic conditions. Echinacea will increase suppuration and care should be taken when using it for problems such as tooth abscesses as it may increase their size and swelling. In this situation it should be taken with detoxifying herbs such as Marigold. Traditionally, Echinacea was used by Plains Indians as 'a remedy for more ailments than any other plant'. The Comanches used the roots for toothache and sore throat, the Sioux for rabies, snakebite and septic conditions. It was also used to treat fits, stomach cramps, enlarged glands, such as mumps, eczema and ulcerous conditions.

COMBINATIONS
With Garlic for throat and chest infections
With Sage and Ginger for gastroenteritis
With St John's Wort for viral infections, especially herpetic infections

16 | *Sambacus Nigra* – ELDERFLOWER
•••••••••••••••••••••••••••••••

Family: *Caprifoliaceae*

Habitat and cultivation
The Elder tree thrives in damp woods, hedges and waste ground, being a European native. The creamy white flowes are harvested in early summer as they open, the berries are picked when ripe in the autumn.

CONSTITUENTS – Flowers:
Flavonoids up to 3% – rutin
Phenolic acids; Triterpenes
Sterols; Volatile oil up to 0.2%
Mucilage; Tannins; Minerals. [Cyanogenic glycosides (leaves only)]

Actions: Diaphoretic, diuretic, anti-inflammatory.

Pharmacology/Research
A poorly researched plant Elderflower has an established diaphoretic effect, though even this is not fully understood. Recent research has indicated that the flowers reduce inflammation. A trial in Israel in 1996 confirmed that Elderberries speed up recovery from the common cold. The berries contain significant levels of anthocyanins and are strongly antioxidant. Like Bilberry they will be helpful in supporting the capillary circulation and are likely to be beneficial for the eyes and eyesight.

Cautions: Elderflowers and berries have no known side effects.

Parts used: Flowers and berries.

PREPARATIONS – Flowers:
Infusion – up to 12g [Berries – up to 25g a day]
Capsules – up to 5g a day
Tincture (1:5) 25% – up to 10ml a day

Key indications: Upper respiratory tract infections – colds; sinusitis; influenza; upper respiratory tract catarrh; fevers; hay fever; coughs.

Indications
Elderflowers make an ideal home treatment for coughs, colds and flus, cooling and lowering fevers. A good diaphoretic it increases elimination via the skin and balances the circulation. The flowers astringe and tone up the mucus membranes of the nose and throat, improving resistance to infection, irritation and allergy. The infusion is soothing and relaxing and produces mild perspiration, and is useful for chronic catarrh and allergies. The infusion taken for 3-4 months before the onset of the hay-fever season can help to reduce the severity of attacks, though Elderflowers may not be sufficient treatment on their own. Elderflowers make a useful remedy for ear infections in children and adults, especially when combined with Echinacea. They can be used in arthritic conditions – by stimulating urine production and sweating, they encourage the removal

of waste products which may cause arthritic symptoms. Elderflower water or the simple infusion may be used to whiten the skin and to remove freckles. The berries are rich in Vitamin C, have traditionally been used for rheumatism, and could be helpful in improving eyesight. They are mildly laxative, but are sufficiently astringent to be useful for diarrhoea as well. As indicated in the research above the berries make an excellent decoction for colds and minor respiratory infections.

COMBINATIONS
With Yarrow and Peppermint for fevers and influenza type infections
With Echinacea and Thyme for ear infections
With Nettle for hay fever

17 | *Inula Helenium* – ELECAMPANE
●●●●●●●●●●●●●●●●●●●●●●●●●●●●●●

Family: *Compositae*

Habitat
Native to southeastern Europe and west Asia. Elecampane is found widely throughout temperate regions.

CONSTITUENTS
Essential oil up to 4% – alantol
Sesquiterpene lactones including – alantolactone
Triterpene saponins – dammaranedienol
Sterols
Polyacetylenes
Inulin up to 44%

Key actions: Expectorant, soothes cough, stimulates sweating, mild bitter, counters intestinal worms.

Pharmacology/Research
Inulin, present in the roots of many Daisy family members, was first isolated from Inula in 1804. Though inulin is mucilaginous and soothes irritation within the chest, the herb as a whole has a stimulant effect encouraging the coughing up of phlegm. The essential oil is partly responsible for this action, being also antiseptic, notably in tuberculosis. Alantolactone is anti-inflammatory, reduces mucus secretions and stimulates the immune system.

Cautions: Occasional allergic skin reactions, if used locally. Contra-indicated in pregnancy and lactation.

Parts used: Root.

PREPARATIONS
Decoction – up to 8g a day
Capsules up to 5g a day
Tincture (1:5) – up to 15ml per week

Key indications: Acute and chronic bronchitis and other chest infections; bronchial asthma; influenza; pleurisy; chronic cough; convalescence; indigestion.

Indications
Elecampane is warming and tonic for both the digestion and the respiratory system, valuable for chest infections, and chronic bronchitis. Its warming effect on the lungs, combined with its ability to gently stimulate expectoration, makes it a safe remedy for the young and the old. It can be prescribed in almost all chesty conditions helping particularly where the patient is *debilitated* – its balance of stimulation and soothing of the lower respiratory mucosa, combined with its mild bitterness improving digestive (especially gastric) secretions and the absorption of nutrients, leads to its specific application in chronic bronchitis and bronchial asthma. It was formerly much used to treat tuberculosis, and combines well with other antiseptic herbs e.g. Thyme and Garlic in treating e.g. influenza, tonsillitis, pneumonia – its restorative, tonic aspect complimenting its antiseptic and fever lowering activity. For the

digestion, it may be taken to stimulate appetite, for dyspepsia, and is a useful remedy for threadworms in children.

COMBINATIONS
With Cayenne, Garlic and Thyme for bronchitis and chest infections in general
With Golden Seal and Elderflower for catarrh
With Liquorice, Lobelia, and Thyme for bronchial asthma

18 | *Tanacetum Parthenium, Chrysanthemum Parthenium* – FEVERFEW

Family: *Compositae*

Habitat and cultivation
Originally from south eastern Europe, Feverfew is now common throughout Europe and North America, thriving in almost any type of soil but preferring a well-drained site. It may be grown from seed, from cuttings or by dividing the rootstock. It is harvested in summer when in flower, while the leaves may be picked as long as they remain healthy.

CONSTITUENTS
Volatile oil – alpha-pinene
Sesquiterpene lactones – parthenolide
Sesquiterpenes – camphor
Acetylenes (in root)

Actions: Analgesic, febrifuge, antirheumatic, emmenagogue.

Pharmacology/Research
After detailed clinical trials in the 1980's in Nottingham, Feverfew is now largely accepted as an effective remedy for migraine. As is often the case

with medicinal plants however, despite this extensive research the exact method of action is not understood. It appears to inhibit the release of serotonin (5HT) by platelets within the central nervous system, a hormone implicated in the triggering of migraines. Parthenolide in particular is credited with this activity. Its effectiveness in the treatment of rheumatoid arthritis has not been confirmed though there are indications that it inhibits prostaglandin production and may therefore be of value in inflammatory arthritic conditions.

Cautions: Feverfew can cause mouth ulcers, a sore tongue and indigestion in a small number of people, though in clinical trials those taking a placebo reported more side effects than those taking Feverfew. Not to be taken during pregnancy.

Parts used: Herb; Leaves.

PREPARATIONS
Fresh leaves – 2-3 leaves in a piece of bread!
Capsules – 125mg a day.

Key indications: Migraine, headache, arthritic and rheumatic pain.

Indications
Feverfew is another herb where recent medical research has confirmed an aspect of its traditional therapeutic use. In this case the wife of a Welsh doctor who cured her 50-year history of migraines with a 10-month course of Feverfew led to detailed scientific investigation. Feverfew should be used in small quantities as a preventative treatment for migraines and at the first signs of an impending migraine attack. It works best when taken *before* the onset of a migraine and is unlikely to bring significant relief once a migraine has set in. It is particularly valuable in migraines associated with the menstrual cycle. The fresh leaves – usually 1-3 in total – are traditionally eaten in a piece of folded bread. Feverfew can be helpful in arthritic and rheumatic pain, especially in combination (see below). The herb has long been used for indigestion, headache and rheumatism, but its major traditional use has always been as a woman's herb. It is a

strong emmenagogue – helping to bring on delayed menstruation – and has been used in this way at least since Roman times. During difficult births it may be used to stimulate the expulsion of the placenta. Surprisingly for a herb with such a name its application in fevers has not really carried through to the present day. The infusion, applied as a lotion makes an effective insect repellent. The closing remarks on Feverfew should be left to John Hill MD in *The Family Herbal* (1772), who states 'In the worst headache this herb exceeds whatever else is known'.

COMBINATIONS
With Willow Bark for inflammatory joint pain and headache

19 | *Allium Sativum* – GARLIC
• •

Family: *Liliaceae*

Habitat and cultivation
Originally from central Asia, Garlic is now cultivated world-wide for use as a food and medicine. Cultivated Garlic is propagated by dividing the bulb into its 'cloves' and planting, preferably in a rich, moist, sandy soil.

CONSTITUENTS
Volatile oil – alliin (0.24% of total weight), alliinase, allicin – methyl allyl sulphides, ajoene: breakdown products
Scordinins
Selenium
Germanium
Glucokinins
Vitamins A, B, C and E

Key actions: Antibiotic, expectorant, diaphoretic, hypotensive, anti-thrombotic, antidiabetic, vermifuge.

Pharmacology/Research

Garlic has been more thoroughly researched than almost any other medicinal plant, though its mode of action has not been fully established – there is still uncertainty about what is responsible for its natural antibiotic activity. Most attention focuses on alliin within the fresh bulb, broken down by alliinase into allicin when the clove is crushed. Allicin and many other constituents of the volatile oil are highly antiseptic and antibiotic, confirming Garlic's use in infections, even severe infections such as dysentery and tuberculosis. Clinical trials have confirmed its ability to lower blood lipid levels, and to lower blood pressure in those with high blood pressure. In vitro experiments with rat aorta tissue showed that Garlic exerts a vasodilatory effect on the endothelium of the artery. Aged cloves have greater anti- oxidant activity than normal garlic – as with the other antiseptic activity this is thought to be largely due to the sulphur mercaptan bridge.

Cautions: Should only be given in small quantities to children.

Parts used: Bulb – the individual 'cloves' are crushed or chopped.

PREPARATIONS

Fresh cloves/bulbs – in food and as an infusion – up to 3 cloves a day
Tincture - rarely used
Tablets or Capsules – dosage as recommended

Key indications: For almost all cardiovascular problems including high blood pressure, raised cholesterol levels, to reduce blood viscosity; in angina, arteriosclerosis, varicosity and prophylactic treatment of strokes. For gum and tooth abscesses, and sore throats – open a capsule, or peel a clove, and crush it gently between the teeth, and hold in place in the cheek adjacent to the site of infection. NB. this can burn the lining of the cheek, though the chances of achieving significant therapeutic improvement are good. For digestive and bronchial infection.

Indications

Garlic is an excellent remedy for chesty conditions and bronchitis, actively countering infection in the lungs and airways – take regularly. It is good for colds, flus and ear infections and reduces catarrh. Digestive infections respond well to Garlic provided it can be kept down. It will improve resistance and recovery in gastroenteritis and can be effective treatment for intestinal parasites. An unbroken clove can be inserted in to the anus to help with threadworms in children. Garlic is a vitally important medicine for the circulation, having both a protective and preventative action against many circulatory disorders. It protects against strokes by inhibiting platelet aggregation, increasing blood thinning activity, reducing fibrinogen levels and blood viscosity and lowering cholesterol levels. It also lowers blood pressure. Lastly, Garlic is anti-fungal, and should always be used as part of treatment for chronic infections, especially where candidiasis is suspected. It can be used alongside conventional antibiotics to support their action and to reduce the occurrence of side effects such as diarrhoea and thrush. It appears to encourage the regrowth of beneficial gut flora. Garlic has always been esteemed as a medicine, with much folklore and superstition attached to it. It is recorded that Garlic was provided in large quantities to labourers building the pyramids in ancient Egypt around 4,500BC. Until the development of penicillin and other antibiotic drugs Garlic was a first line treatment for all manner of infections – from tuberculosis to typhoid. It was used by the ton to dress wounds in the trenches of the First World War, and still makes an excellent antiseptic dressing for wounds and ulcerous sores.

COMBINATIONS
With Hawthorn for high blood pressure
With Ginger for digestive infections
With Echinacea for viral, and chronic, infections

20 | *Gentiana Lutea* – GENTIAN
•••••••••••••••••••••••••••

Family: *Gentianacea*

Habitat and cultivation

The largest member of this diverse family Gentian is native to the Alps and other mountainous regions of central and southern Europe between altitudes of 700-2400m. It flourishes in Alpine meadows but occurs from Spain to the Balkans. The large root crowns can be split or it can be readily grown from seed, needing a loamy soil and sheltered position. The root is dug up in the early autumn and dried.

CONSTITUENTS
Bitter principles – gentiopicroside, amarogentin
Loigosaccharides – gentianose
Polysaccharides – inulin
Xanthones; Phenolic acids; Pectin

Key actions: Bitter, digestive stimulant, stomachic.

Pharmacology/Research

The bitter principles within Gentian stimulate bitter taste receptors on the tongue causing a reflex increase in the production of saliva and gastric secretions, and stimulation of the appetite. Although present in much smaller quantities than gentiopicroside, amarogentin is largely responsible for the bitterness of Gentian being 5,000 times more bitter than gentiopicroside and tasted at dilutions of 1:50,000. It is possibly the most bitter substance on the planet!

Other species: All the Gentian family are bitter tasting plants and many have been used in herbal medicine as a result e.g. *Gentiana scabrae* (Japanese Gentian).

Cautions: Avoid in cases of strongly acid indigestion, and peptic ulceration.

47

Parts used: Root.

PREPARATIONS
Tincture (1:5) 45% – generally as 10-20 drops before meals three times a day
Bitters such as Angostura Bitters are made with Gentian and can be used in a similar way

Key indications: Digestive weakness and underactivity particularly of the stomach; to aid digestion and absorption of nutrients.

Indications
Gentian stimulates stomach activity and relieves symptoms linked to weak digestion, wind, indigestion, poor appetite, and failure to gain weight. Stomach and other secretions are increased leading to improved absorption of nutrients, e.g. iron, vit B12. A 'pure' bitter, Gentian is useful in almost any case of poor digestive tone, involving deficient digestive secretions, and reduced or impaired absorption. It is particularly useful for iron deficiency anaemia and is often added in small quantities to prescriptions for heavy menstrual bleeding and in other situations where blood loss has occurred. Liver and gall bladder activity is also stimulated. In summary, Gentian is the remedy for underactive digestive states and an atrophic digestive system (thus its greater use in the elderly). The name Gentian attests to its ancient use in classical times, Gentius being a King of Illyria in the 2nd century BC who reputedly discovered the virtues of the plant.

COMBINATIONS
With Ginger to stimulate appetite

21 | *Zingiber Officinalis* – GINGER
•••••••••••••••••••••••••••

Family: *Zinzigiberaceae*

Habitat and cultivation
A native of tropical Asia but now widely grown throughout the tropics, Ginger is cultivated from division of the rootstock. It flourishes in fertile soils and needs a good rainfall. The roots are dug up when the plant is 10 months old, washed soaked and sometimes boiled and peeled.

CONSTITUENTS
Volatile oil 1–3% – zingiberene 20–30%
Oleoresin 4–7.5% – gingerols, shogaols (mainly when dried)

Actions: Anti-emetic, carminative, spasmolytic, circulatory stimulant, antitussive, anti–inflammatory, antiseptic.

Pharmacology/Research
A well researched herb, Ginger has been shown to be highly effective for travel sickness and nausea. One trial (at Bart's Hospital in Anaethesia 45 [1990]) found Ginger to be more effective than conventional treatments in relieving post-operative nausea. In a Chinese trial, 70% of patients recovered when given Ginger for bacillary dysentery. The established therapeutic benefits of Ginger are largely due to the essential oil content and the oleoresins. Gingerol is highly acrid and responsible for much of the pungency and circulatory stimulation. NB. The shogaols are formed in the plant on drying, and are more strongly irritant and acrid than the constituents present in the fresh rhizome.

Cautions: None.

Parts used: Root (rhizome) – fresh or dried.

PREPARATIONS
Infusion – NB difference between fresh and dried root. Both excellent for domestic use
Capsule – up to a max of 2g a day
Tincture (1:2) – up to 1.5ml a day

Key indications: Common cold, nausea, vomiting and dyspepsia, bronchitis, poor peripheral circulation and chilblains, prevention of stroke, migraine.

Indications

Ginger is strongly carminative and antiseptic within the gastro-intestinal tract, and is a key herb for stomach and gut infections, such as food poisoning, and dysentery. It is also specific for indigestion due to infection or weak gastric function, and for nausea whether due to morning sickness, travel sickness, or after operative anaesthesia. For morning sickness and travel sickness capsules are ideal. Ginger is commonly used for upper and lower respiratory tract infections – coughs, colds, flus, bronchitis and whooping cough, and as with digestive problems, warms and soothes the affected area. Combine with Garlic for digestive infections, and with Garlic and Echinacea for respiratory infection. Like all 'heating' herbs Ginger stimulates the circulation, especially to the *periphery*. Used therefore to improve perfusion (and encourage sweating) to the skin, head, and periphery in general. It helps to lower body temperature in fever, and is a valuable remedy for managing high fevers. Its warming action also makes it useful for chilblains, poor circulation to the hands and feet, for certain skin problems (not eczema), while its antioxidant and anti-blood clotting aspects make it a herb of choice for preventing stroke. In Chinese herbal medicine the fresh and dried roots are treated as different remedies – the fresh being more subtle and used for chills, fevers, headache and aching muscles, while the dried root is used more for 'internal' cold, with cold hands, weak pulse and pale complexion.

COMBINATIONS
With Chamomile for nausea, vomiting and dyspepsia
With Garlic for digestive infections
With Echinacea and/or Garlic for respiratory infection such as bronchitis
With Capsicum for chilblains
With Ginkgo as a prophylactic for stroke

22 | *Ginkgo Biloba* – GINKGO
•••••••••••••••••••••••••

Family: *Gingkoaceae*

Habitat and cultivation
Native to China, though no longer found growing wild, the Ginkgo tree is cultivated commercially in large scale plantations in China, in France near Bordeaux and in South Carolina, USA. The leaves are harvested in the autumn.

CONSTITUENTS
Flavone glycosides
Ginkgolides (diterpenes)
Bilobalide (sesquiterpene)

Key actions: Circulatory stimulant and tonic, anti-asthmatic, anti-spasmodic, anti-inflammatory, anti-allergenic.

Pharmacology/Research
Since the 1960's extensive research and over 50 clinical trials have established that Ginkgo has great therapeutic value in poor cerebral circulation, thus improving memory, concentration and aiding in cases of dementia – both Alzheimer's and multi-infarct dementia. Originally it was thought that the flavone glycosides were responsible for its effectiveness in improving poor cerebral and peripheral blood flow, but it became clear that this was not the sole factor involved. Ginkgo, and the ginkgolides in particular, inhibits Platelet Activating Factor (PAF), which causes platelet aggregation and inflammatory and allergenic changes, and is implicated in a wide range of problems including asthma, urticaria and psoriasis. Ginkgo extract however acts synergistically and is *more* effective in this respect than any of its individual constituents. The bilobide content has a potent nerve protective action against ischaemic damage (damage caused by insufficient blood flow). A French study in 1993 indicated that Ginkgo standardised extract relieved severe pre-menstrual breast tenderness.

Cautions: Ginkgo, and its standardised extract, has been shown to be extremely free from side effects.

Parts used: Leaves.

PREPARATIONS

Decoction/powder/capsule – up to 5g a day in three divided doses

Key indications: Cerebral vascular insufficiency; peripheral vascular insufficiency including intermittent claudication; dementia; depression; neuralgia and neuropathy; asthma; multiple sclerosis.

Indications
Thought to be the oldest tree on the planet, interest has focused on Ginkgo's remarkable ability to improve the circulation, especially poor circulation to the brain. It has become a best selling medicine in France and Germany being taken daily by millions of people from middle age onwards to maintain or improve cerebral circulation, memory and concentration and to reduce the possibility of a stroke. It is probably the most useful herbal medicine in the treatment of dementia, and has value as an anti-depressant (see combinations below). Ginkgo is also a tonic herb and many people feel an increased sense of vitality and mental well-being when taking Ginkgo. Its other potential indications within the central nervous system include prevention of stroke and thrombus formation, tinnitus, vertigo, dizziness, sudden onset nerve deafness, nerve pain and nerve disease in general e.g. multiple sclerosis. Ginkgo improves the circulation as a whole – and is therefore useful in arteriosclerosis, intermittent claudication and ischaemic heart disease; its anti-inflammatory and anti- allergenic activity makes it useful in a range of other conditions, notably asthma, and it may be potentially valuable in conditions as varied as psoriasis, auto-immune problems, and organ transplants. As indicated above Ginkgo has proved useful for pre-menstrual problems and combines well with Agnus Castus for pre-menstrual syndrome, especially where breast tenderness and swelling are a key factor.

COMBINATIONS
With Hawthorn for ischaemic heart disease and peripheral ischaemia
With Agnus Castus for pre-menstrual syndrome
With St John's Wort for depression, neuralgia and nerve disorders
With Black Cohosh for tinnitus
With Ginger to reduce risk of stroke

23 | *Panax Ginseng*
GINSENG (Chinese: Ren Shen)
•••••••••••••••••••••••••••••

Family: *Araliaceae*

Habitat and cultivation
Native to north east China and Russia, and North Korea. Extremely rare in the wild. Root of wild and cultivated plants are very different in quality. The plant takes 4 years to mature; cultivation requires great skill. Cultivated in Korea since 1300.

CONSTITUENTS
Steroidal saponins – ginsenosides 0.7-3% – at least 25 have been identified
Acetylenic compounds
Panaxans
Sesquiterpenes

Actions: Adaptogen, stimulant, tonic.

Pharmacology/Research
Ginseng has been researched in depth over the past 20-30 years, and its remarkable 'adaptogenic' quality – supporting the body in coping with stress, fatigue and exhaustion, has been more than confirmed. The capacity to adapt to extremes of temperature, hunger, and mental and

emotional stress is significantly improved, while when sleep, rather than stimulation, is required by the body Ginseng will produce a sedative response. The ginsenosides are responsible for much of this activity and stimulate release of ACTH from the pituitary gland. Ginseng also increases non-specific immune function, and therefore resistance to infection, and supports liver function.

Other species: Other species also have significant therapeutic benefits – notably American Ginseng (*Panax quinquefolium*), and *Panax pseudoginseng.*

Cautions: Side effects such as high blood pressure and sleeplessness are associated only with an excessive intake. Avoid caffeine and caffeine drinks while taking Ginseng. For the young and healthy, take for no more than 6 weeks at a time. Contraindicated during pregnancy, while breastfeeding, during acute illness and in high blood pressure.

Parts used: Root.

PREPARATIONS
Dried root: chewed/powder/decoction/capsule – up to 2g a day as single dose. Usually start at a lower dosage e.g. 500mg once a day.

Key indications: Physical, environmental and emotional stress; chronic tiredness and infection; impotence; overwork.

Indications
Best known as a stimulant and tonic for athletes and those subject to physical stress, and as an aphrodisiac for men, it is also a remedy for old age, being taken traditionally through the long hard winters of northern and central China by anyone late middle aged and older. In China it is considered to 'quieten the spirit', an indication of its restorative action. Living up to its description as an adaptogen Ginseng will tend to support the body's needs in an *individual* way – so that it acts as a stimulant to those with a strong vitality, and as a tonic, or even sedative to those with a deficient vitality resulting from long term or severe illness or old age.

The range of indications is great – from its 'normal' use to chronic fatigue syndrome, dementia, and HIV/AIDS. Other indications include impotence, chronic exhaustion from long-term stress, headaches/tension associated with overwork and jet lag.

COMBINATIONS
With Ginkgo for overwork and exhaustion
With Damiana for male sexual dysfunction

24 | *Eleutherococcus Senticosus* – SIBERIAN GINSENG
●●●●●●●●●●●●●●●●●●●●●●

Family: *Araliaceae*

Habitat and cultivation
Native to the steppes of eastern Russia, China, Korea, and Japan. Can be grown from seed but is a very difficult plant to germinate.

CONSTITUENTS
Eleutherosides A,B,B$_1$,C,D,E – 0.6-0.9%
Phenylpropanoids
Lignans; coumarins; triterpenoid saponins; sacchaddes including glycans – eleutherans

Key actions: Adaptogen (aids ability to cope with stresses), tonic, stimulant, immune-protector.

Pharmacology/Research
There has been much research into Siberian Ginseng in Russia, though the exact method by which it stimulates stamina and resistance to stress is not understood. It has a marked action on the adrenal glands, helping to withstand heat, cold, infection, other physical stresses, radiation and even

the effects of weightlessness in astronauts. Athletes have experienced up to a 9% improvement in stamina when taking this herb, probably due to improved oxygen metabolism (due perhaps to an increased production of mitochondria). Apart from eleutheroside A, Siberian Ginseng's active constituents are quite different from the saponins found in Ginseng *(Panax ginseng).* Eleutheroside E is thought to be mainly responsible for the increase in resistance to stress. The glycans are immunostimulant when injected but may not be so orally. Though Siberian Ginseng is generally used to promote stamina and resistance, it also stimulates nonspecific immune resistance during illness, including cancer. Additionally, it has an anti-toxic action reducing the effect of toxins and protecting against side-effects from both radiotherapy and chemotherapy.

Cautions: Side effects are rare. Avoid in hypertension. As a simple tonic take for no more than 6 weeks, then rest for at least 2 weeks. Avoid caffeine when taking. Avoid during pregnancy or while breastfeeding.

Parts used: Roots

PREPARATIONS
Decoction – up to 4g a day
Capsules – up to 4g a day, start at 500mg twice a day and increase if required
Tincture (1:5) – up to 75ml per week

Key indications: Aiding adaptation to stress – physical, chemical, emotional etc; chronic fatigue; to improve resistance to infection.

Indications
Since the extensive research carried out in Russia from the 1950s onwards Siberian Ginseng has become commonly used. It is best given for the following: to improve mental and physical performance, e.g. examinations; to reduce the effects of physical stress, e.g. athletic training; to treat prolonged exhaustion, e.g. overwork, long-term stress, etc; to protect against chemo- and other toxicity; to aid recovery/prevent deterioration in acute, and especially, chronic illness, including, e.g.

HIV/AIDS; and as a general tonic helping to improve non-specific immunity and to maintain well-being. In China Siberian Ginseng (known as Wu Jia Pi) is used to treat cold damp conditions.

COMBINATIONS
With Echinacea and Thyme for chronic infection
With St John's Wort for chronic fatigue

25 | *Hydrastis Canadensis* – GOLDEN SEAL

Family: *Ranunculaceae*

Habitat and cultivation
Grows in moist and mountainous woodland areas throughout much of Canada and the United States, preferring soils well covered by dead leaves. Due to excessive collection of the root Hydrastis is no longer common in its natural habitat. It is now cultivated as a medicinal herb but requires an environment very close to its natural habitat to flourish.

CONSTITUENTS
Isoquinoline alkaloids – hydrastine; berberine; canadine
Chlorogenic acid
Resin: Volatile oil

Key actions: Aids bile flow, antimicrobial, tonic, mild laxative, anti-inflammatory, uterine stimulant, stops bleeding, astringent.

Pharmacology/Research
Very little research has been undertaken in to the whole plant – what research there is is into the isoquinoline alkaloids, to which Golden Seal's activity is largely due. Hydrastine is vasoconstrictive and stimulant to the

autonomic nervous system; berberine is bitter, antibacterial, amoebicidal, choleretic and sedative to the central nervous system; canadine is stimulant to the muscles of the womb. The isoquinoline alkaloids and berberine in particular are strongly antibiotic against a number of digestive pathogens e.g. Chlamydia, Salmonella, Shigella, Giardia etc, making Golden Seal an important herbal medicine for enteric infection.

Cautions: Do not take in pregnancy or while breastfeeding; or with high blood pressure. Toxic if taken to excess. Max. 3 months continual use.

Parts used: Rhizome

PREPARATIONS
Decoction/capsules – max 1g a day
Tr (1:5) 60% – up to 5ml a day

Key indications: Catarrhal problems; upper respiratory infections e.g. sinusitis, conjunctivitis; gastro-intestinal infections – giardia, etc; peptic ulceration and inflammatory problems of the digestive system; vaginal and uterine infection; psoriasis.

Indications

Different authorities emphasise different aspects of Golden Seal's therapeutic value. There is however common ground confirming it as a potent remedy for disorders affecting mucus membranes throughout the body, notably in the eye, the ear, nose and throat, the stomach and intestines, and the vagina. Use a dilute lotion as an eyewash, as a mouthwash for infected gums, or as a wash or douche for vaginal thrush and infections. Internally, it increases digestive secretions, astringes the mucus membranes lining the gut, and checks inflammation – do not prescribe for extended periods of time as it is thought to inhibit absorption of nutrients – notably the B vitamins. With a tonic action on the mucus membranes of the digestive tract, respiratory tract and vagina it is valuable in catarrhal states. It aids healing of ulcers, especially peptic ulceration, as well as infective and inflammatory problems throughout the gastrointestinal tract. A strong stimulant of bile production it is used for liver and gall bladder weakness, and to counter gastro-intestinal infections such as amoebic dysentery. The whole herb and the isoquinoline alkaloids in particular are active in reducing the severity of psoriasis. It may be used to reduce heavy menstrual bleeding.

COMBINATIONS
With Liquorice and Chamomile for peptic ulceration and gastritis
With Eyebright and Echinacea for conjunctivitis
With Garlic and Wormwood for digestive infections
With Echinacea, Nettle, and Dandelion root for hay fever

26 | *Crataegus Spp* – HAWTHORN
• •

Family: *Rosaceae*

Habitat and cultivation
Hawthorn grows in hedgerows, copses and fields throughout the British Isles, and all temperate regions of the northern hemisphere. It is generally cultivated from hardwood cuttings. The seed takes 18 months to germinate. The flowers and leaves are harvested in late spring, the berries in late summer.

CONSTITUENTS
Bioflavonoids including – rutin, quercitin
Triterpenoids
Oligomeric pro-cyanidins
Cyanogenic glycosides
Amines – trimethylamine (in flowers)
Polyphenols
Coumarins
Tannins (condensed)

Actions: Cardiotonic, vasodilator, relaxant.

Pharmacology/Research
The bioflavonoids produce arterial vasodilation, and specifically act on the coronary arteries, thus contributing to the overall reduction in symptoms of angina indicated in clinical research. The bioflavonoids and pro-cyanidins are also strongly anti-oxidant, aiding in the prevention of blood vessel degeneration throughout the body. The cyanogenic glycosides are sedative and slow heart rate, encouraging greater heart efficiency. Widely researched in Germany, a recent double blind placebo controlled trial (Schmidt, U. et al in *Phytomedicine* (1994) 1/1 pp 17-24) showed that patients with mild chronic heart failure responded significantly to treatment with a Hawthorn extract; the patients' working capacity as measured by an ergometer bicycle increased markedly; systolic BP and heart rate reduced and clinical symptoms improved. No side effects were observed.

Cautions: No known side effects. Do not take without consulting a medical herbalist or doctor if taking conventional medication for circulatory or heart problems.

Parts used: Flowering tops; Leaves – highest bioflavonoid content; Berries.

PREPARATIONS
Infusion (flowers and leaves) – up to 3g a day
Decoction (berries) – up to 3g a day
Capsule – up to 2g a day
Tincture (1:5) – up to 50ml per week

Key indications: High blood pressure, low blood pressure, angina, mild chronic heart failure, arteriosclerosis, intermittent claudication.

Indications
Hawthorn was traditionally used in Europe for kidney and bladder stones, and as a diuretic, and 16th and 17th century herbals – Gerard, Culpeper

and K'Eogh – all list these uses. A specific for angina, and coronary artery disease; it works well but may take some months to produce notable results. Valuable in high blood pressure, and due to its bioflavonoid content, for athero- and arteriosclerosis. It appears to have a *normalising* effect helping to lower high blood pressure *and* to raise low blood pressure – the clinical experience of herbal practitioners and some research suggests this is the case. As the above research indicates Hawthorn is useful in cases of mild congestive heart failure and irregular heart beat. It may well be thought of as a tonic 'food' for the heart, supporting blood flow through the coronary circuit and thus improving overall heart function, especially where normal function is compromised as in mild heart failure. It has a tonic action on the inner lining of blood vessels in general and can be used in appropriate combination for venous as well as arterial problems.

COMBINATIONS
For mild to moderate heart failure with Gingko and Dandelion leaf
For high blood pressure with Garlic and Valerian

27 | *Piper Methysticum* – KAVA KAVA

Family: *Piperaceae*

Habitat and cultivation
Kava Kava grows throughout Polynesia, the Pacific Islands as far east as Hawaii. The plant is grown entirely from runners, being cultivated commercially in the USA. The root may be harvested at any time of the year.

CONSTITUENTS
Resin containing lactones – kawain
Piperidine alkaloid – pipermethysticine

Actions: Stimulant, tonic, anxiolytic, spasmolytic, diuretic, antiseptic.

Pharmacology/Research
The kava lactones have a depressant effect on the central nervous system and are antispasmodic. Kawain, in particular is sedative, and kawain has been used in Germany as a mild sedative and treatment for epilepsy. The kava lactones also have an anaesthetic effect on the lining of the urinary tubules and bladder. The root produces a narcotic effect in excess. French and German clinical trials have strongly supported the view that Kava Kava is an effective anxiolytic herb with no sedative activity, patients ability to drive or operate machinery was not effected while taking the herb. One German trial showed a significant reduction in anxiety, depression and menopausal problems in women with menopausal symptoms.

Cautions: Safe in moderate dosage, do not take for a prolonged period of time e.g. more than 3 months. Not suitable during pregnancy. Long term consumption or high dosages can cause dry scaly and pigmented skin patches, which however clear once treatment is stopped.

Parts used: Root – traditionally chewed and fermented with saliva.

PREPARATIONS
Decoction – up to 10g a day
Capsule – up to 2.5g a day
Tincture (1:5) – up to 10ml a day

Key indications: Anxiety and nervous tension, insomnia, urinary tract infection.

Indications
Kava Kava's medicinal use is reflected in its traditional ritual use in the South Sea Islands – as a calming, even tranquillising herb that has tonic

and antiseptic properties. Its antiseptic action led it to be considered a specific in treating venereal disease in the past, and though it is no longer commonly used in this way, it is a valuable urinary antiseptic helping to counter urinary infections and to settle an 'irritable' bladder. Kava Kava has tonic, strengthening and mildly analgesic properties and is valuable in treating chronic pain, reducing sensitivity and relaxing muscles tensed in the protective response to pain. Combined with its cleansing diuretic action, this often makes it beneficial in arthritic problems such as gout, where symptomatic relief of pain is supported by removal of waste products. Taken in quantity the tonic and calming effect of the herb produces an euphoric state, probably why it has long been considered an aphrodisiac. Despite its largely non-sedative action it may be helpful in mild insomnia.

COMBINATIONS
With Valerian in anxiety and insomnia
With Cornsilk for chronic cystitis and irritable bladder

28 | *Melissa Officinalis* – LEMON BALM

Family: *Lamiacae*

Habitat and cultivation
Though native to southern Europe Lemon Balm is now found throughout the world. The herb should be harvested in the summer as the flowers begin to open, when they have the maximum concentration of volatile oil. The herb needs to be dried quickly but carefully, and the fresh herb is often preferable.

CONSTITUENTS
Volatile oil – 0.1-0.2% – citral, caryophyllene oxide, linalool, citronellal
Flavonoids; Polyphenols including glycosides of caffeic and rosmarinic acids
Triterpenes; Tannins

Key actions: Relaxant, anti-spasmodic, diaphoretic, carminative, anti-viral, tonic.

Pharmacology/Research
Lemon Balm owes much of its relaxant and mildly tranquillising activity to its volatile oil, especially citral and citronellal. Though present in very small quantities the volatile oil is also responsible for the herb's significant anti-spasmodic activity – comparable in strength to papaverine from the Opium Poppy (*Papaver somniferum*). The polyphenols (which are present in relatively large amounts) and tannins are strongly anti-viral, and are extremely effective against the herpes viruses, especially herpes simplex which produces cold sores. One German study showed that compared to conventional treatments the average healing time of cold sores was halved to about 5 days, and the time between outbreaks doubled. To achieve greatest effect however, the herb must be used in the early stages of infection. The herb inhibits thyroid function. Preliminary research (1995/ongoing) in Newcastle suggests the fresh herb and oil may be of potential use in treating Alzheimer's disease.

Cautions: Avoid in low thyroid function.

Parts used: Herb.

PREPARATIONS
Infusion – up to 15g a day
Capsules – up to 3g a day
Tincture (1:5) – up to 15ml a day
Cream/ointment – topically

Key indications: Anxiety, nervous palpitations, nervous indigestion, headache, migraine, low spirits, cold sores.

Indications

Lemon Balm is a tonic herb, revivifying and lifting the spirits, and predisposing it is thought, to a long and healthy life. Other traditional uses include healing wounds – the juice being preferred here, relieving palpitations and 'relaxing' the heart. Many of these uses are still current, and the herb is prescribed for anxiety, mild depression, restlessness and irritability, reducing feelings of nervousness and panic. It will often quieten a racing heart, and is a valuable remedy for nervous palpitations. It may be taken where acute or chronic anxiety is interfering in normal digestive activity, e.g. indigestion, acidity, bloating, colic and peptic ulcer, combining well with Chamomile here. The herb will help in headache, migraine and dizziness, though it is best used in combination for these conditions. In view of its anti-thyroid effect Melissa is indicated for hyperthyroid states, though it will have little or no effect in severe cases. Apply as a lotion, cream or ointment to herpes sores – at the earliest signs of infection.

COMBINATIONS
With Limeflowers for palpitations and panic attacks
With St John's Wort and Echinacea for cold sores
With St John's Wort and Rosemary in depression

29 | *Tilia Platyphyllos or Cordata* – LIMEFLOWERS or LINDEN FLOWERS
●●●

Family: *Tiliaceae*

Habitat and cultivation

A common native European tree found growing wild, but often found growing in urban environments, especially in avenues lining roads and carriageways. The flowers with their bracts are collected in the summer.

FIFTY VITAL HERBS

CONSTITUENTS
Flavonoids – mainly quercetin and kaempferol glycosides
Caffeic and other acids; mucilage; tannins
Volatile oil (0.02%-0.1%); traces of benzodiazepene-like compounds

Key actions: Diaphoretic, relaxant, anxiolytic, antispasmodic, lowers blood pressure, mild demulcent.

Pharmacology/Research
Recent Argentinian research suggests that Limeflowers (*Tilia tomentosa*) may have an anxiolytic activity similar to that of benzodiazepenes such as Valium, which would confirm the traditional use of the herb as a sedative and relaxant. The high flavonoid content makes it a valuable medicine for anteriosclerosis and circulatory disorders. The herb is thought to have an antispasmodic activity.

Cautions: none known, though it has been reported that excessive use may result in cardiac toxicity.

Parts used: Flowers/bracts

PREPARATIONS
Infusion – up to 10g a day
Capsule – up to 5g a day
Tincture (1:5) 45% – up to 20ml a day

Key indications: Tension headache, migraine, anxiety and stress, nervous palpitations, colds and flu, upper respiratory catarrh, coughs, high blood pressure, arteriosclerosis.

Indications
Relaxing, diaphoretic and sedative, Limeflowers are the herb of choice for tension and sinus headaches, helping to ease congestion, clear associated headache and 'fogginess' and encourage sleep. It is an excellent remedy for stress and panic, often used in conjunction with Lemon Balm and/or Valerian for anxiety, headaches and nervous palpitations. It is also used for

66

migraine and vertigo. The flowers seem to have a predilection for the head and bring relief to colds and 'flus, checking nasal cararrh formation and reducing fever. Limeflowers are commonly taken to lower high blood pressure, particularly where this is due to emotional factors, and is used long term to treat high systolic blood pressure associated with arteriosclerosis – their long term use aiding the tone of blood vessel walls. It is surprisingly emollient applied to the skin and is traditionally used as a lotion for itchy skin in France.

COMBINATIONS
With Lemon Balm for anxiety and nervous palpitations
With Valeria for high blood pressure associated with nervous tension
With Elderflower or berry for head colds

30 | *Glycyrrhiza Glabra* – LIQUORICE
• •

Family: *Leguminoseae*

Habitat and cultivation
Liquorice grows wild in southeastern Europe, and south-west Asia. It prefers a sandy soil, proximity to water, and a warm climate. The roots are divided and planted in the spring. Harvesting of the root does not take place until the 3rd or 4th year in autumn.

CONSTITUENTS
Triterpene saponins – glycyrrhizic acid (up to 6%)
Flavonoids; Polysaccharides; Sterols; Coumarins; Asparagin

Key actions: Anti-inflammatory, expectorant, demulcent, adrenal tonic, mild laxative, oestrogenic, anti-viral.

Pharmacology/Research
Liquorice and in particular glycyrrhizic acid (on hydolysis in the gut) has a strong anti-inflammatory and anti-arthritic action similar to hydrocortisone and other cortico-steroids. It reduces the breakdown of these steroids within the liver and kidneys, thereby increasing their activity within the body. It reduces stomach secretions but acts to produce a thick protective mucus coating for the lining of the stomach. Though glycyrrhizic acid increases fluid retention within the body (it inhibits metabolism of aldosterone) and has a hypertensive effect (raises blood pressure), asparagin is a strong diuretic counterbalancing this effect within the remedy as a whole (the root has traditionally been considered to be a diuretic). Glycyrrhizic acid is 50 times sweeter than sugar. Glycyrrhizin (= 1 molecule of glycyrrhizic acid and 2 molecules glucoronic acid) stimulates interferon production, research in Japan (Hikino in Economic and Medicinal Plant Research vol 1, 1985) confirming this activity. It has been shown to be effective in the treatment of chronic hepatitis and liver cirrhosis; it also inhibits prostaglandin formation.

Cautions: Do not take in high blood pressure; potassium deficiency (or if taking diuretics or drugs for heart treatment); acute or chronic renal disease; and pregnancy.

Parts used: Root – can be chewed raw or dried.

PREPARATIONS
Decoction – rarely if ever used on its own: 1-4g up to three times a day
Capsules – up to 2.5g a day
Fluid extract (1:1) – up to 30ml pw

Key indications: Peptic ulcer and other inflammatory states of the digestive system; bronchitis; rheumatoid and osteo-arthritis; hepatitis; eczema.

Indications

A powerful anti-inflammatory for digestive, respiratory, rheumatic and skin disorders, an anti-viral remedy, and a restorative for the adrenal cortex, Liquorice is one of the most important and pleasant tasting medicinal plants of all. It is indicated in a wide range of inflammatory conditions affecting the digestion e.g. stomatitis, gastritis, peptic ulceration, and excessive acid production; in many respiratory conditions – asthma, bronchitis, dry coughs; in arthritis: and in some inflammatory skin problems e.g. psoriasis. It has a strongly supportive effect upon the adrenal glands, helping in Addison's disease and, as significantly, aiding in withdrawal from hydrocortisone treatment – it appears to stimulate adrenal cortex function, which is inhibited by artificially raised hydrocortisone levels. It also has a place in the treatment of chronic fatigue syndrome and other problems where systemic exhaustion is a feature. Liquorice is hepatoprotective and in view of its ability to stimulate interferon production has a place in the treatment of hepatitis A, B and C. Due to its oestrogenic activity it is of value during the menopause, being used traditionally in Russian herbal medicine for hot flushes and other menopausal problems. Liquorice has a gentle laxative action. Topically it is soothing for inflamed eyes. It is a useful remedy to include in many prescriptions, and is considered a 'unifying' herb in traditional Chinese medicine. It is hard to think of a prescription where it would be completely out of place.

COMBINATIONS

With Chamomile, Golden Seal and Slippery Elm for peptic ulcer
With Milk Thistle, Echinacea and Golden Seal for hepatitis
With Sage and Wild Yam for menopausal problems
With Elecampane and Thyme for bronchitis and cough

31 | *Lobelia Inflata* – LOBELIA, Indian Tobacco
•••

Family: *Campanulaceae*

Habitat and cultivation
A common weed throughout the eastern United States, Lobelia grows on roadsides and in neglected areas. It is harvested in the autumn when after flowering and needs to be carefully dried.

CONSTITUENTS
Piperidine alkaloids – principally lobeline, but many others present; Carboxylic acids

Key actions: Respiratory stimulant, antispasmodic, expectorant, emetic (causes vomiting), diaphoretic.

Pharmacology/Research
The piperidine alkaloids, and lobeline in particular, have a similar pharmacological activity to nicotine so that Lobelia may be used to aid withdrawal from tobacco addiction. The alkaloids reflexly stimulate the respiratory centre within the brain stem producing stronger and deeper breathing. As the alkaloids are quickly broken down within the body the herb is often more effective when applied topically, or as a suppository, or taken sublingually as drops of tincture. The whole plant is strongly antispasmodic. Traditionally known as Puke Weed, Lobelia stimulates the vomiting centre in the medulla oblongata, and at more than low doses is an effective emetic.

Other species: A number of different species have been used by native Americans; one *L. syphilitica* (Great Lobelia) as its name suggests was credited with powers to cure and treat syphilis by Indians and white settlers alike. A Chinese species *Lobelia chinensis* is used in traditional Chinese medicine as a diuretic and in the treatment of snake bite.

Cautions: Toxic in overdosage, but so strongly emetic that vomiting will normally result from more than small doses preventing excessive absorption.

Parts used: Leaves.

PREPARATIONS
Capsules and tablets – take as recommended on label
Inhaled smoke – traditional North American use for symptomatic relief of asthma

Key indications: Asthma, bronchial asthma, bronchitis, catarrh of the upper or lower respiratory tract, difficulty in breathing, withdrawal from tobacco; topically – muscle spasm.

Indications
A powerful antispasmodic and respiratory stimulant, Lobelia is a valuable remedy for asthma, especially bronchial asthma, and bronchitis. By relaxing the muscles of the small bronchial tubes it opens up the airways. At the same time it stimulates breathing and expectoration (increases coughing up of phlegm). These are the most common uses for Lobelia – almost always in combination with other respiratory herbs such as Thyme and Elecampane. In the North American Physiomedicalist tradition Lobelia is always combined with Cayenne Pepper, the hot stimulant action of Cayenne pushing the circulation into areas which have been relaxed by Lobelia e.g. the chest. This combination also leads to improved central and peripheral blood flow, supporting the system as a whole during acute illness. Lobelia is often most effective when applied topically to the skin to relieve aching or tense muscles or muscles that have gone 'rock hard' trying to protect painful joints. It may also be taken internally, usually with Cramp Bark to ease muscle sprains, and back and arthritic problems where muscle tension is a key factor. Lobelia's medicinal use was championed by Samuel Thompson, the pioneering early 19th century American herbalist, who made Lobelia the mainstay of his therapeutics – generally using it as an emetic to induce vomiting, cleanse the stomach of its contents and prevent fermentation during fever.

COMBINATIONS
With Liquorice and Thyme for asthma
With Elecampane and Echinacea for bronchitis
With Cramp Bark for muscle tension
With Valerian for tobacco withdrawal

32 | *Calendula Officinalis* – MARIGOLD, POT MARIGOLD
●●●●●●●●●●●●●●●●●●●●●●●●●●●●●

Family: *Compositae*

Habitat and cultivation
Native to southern Europe but grown as a garden plant in temperate regions around the world. Easily grown from seed, flourishes in almost all soils. Prefers a sunny site. The flowers are harvested on opening from June onwards and dried in the shade (up to 35°C).

CONSTITUENTS
Triterpenoid saponins
Resins
Bitter glycosides; Essential oil; Sterols; Flavonoids; Mucilage

Key actions: Anti-inflammatory, wound healer, antispasmodic, anti-haemorrhagic, antiseptic, stimulates sweating, stimulates onset of menstruation.

Pharmacology/Research
Marigold has been shown to have antiseptic properties, though its ability to counter infection appears to be wider than this – it has constituents which are anti-fungal (the resins especially), anti-bacterial and anti-viral.

It appears to astringe (tighten up) capillaries, explaining its therapeutic effectiveness in cuts, wounds and inflammatory conditions. It is one of the few herbs which is astringent but has a low tannin content, the astringency being due to the resins.

Cautions: None

Parts used: Flowerheads

PREPARATIONS
Infusion – up to 25g a day if required
Capsule – generally 1–3g a day
Fixed Oil – not normally used internally; a good base oil for application to the skin
Ointment/Cream – easily made at home or commonly available over the counter

Key indications: Internally: Inflammatory disorders of the digestive system; infection or congestion of the lymphatic system; painful and irregular periods. Externally: Healing inflamed and sore rashes/wounds/cuts/grazes etc; fungal skin infections (with Ti-tree oil); vaginal infections.

Indications

A herb for the skin – providing effective treatment for most minor skin problems. Use for cuts, grazes and wounds; for red and inflamed skin generally, including minor burns and sunburn; for acne and many rashes; and for fungal conditions such as ringworm, athlete's foot and thrush (other anti-fungals may be more effective e.g. Ti-tree oil, Thyme). Use for nappy rash and cradle cap in babies, and to soothe sore nipples, especially when breastfeeding (oil or ointment). The flowers or petals may be used as a poultice for sore breasts and mastitis. Add essential oils such as German Chamomile up to 2.5% maximum as required. Taken internally the flowers/petals are indicated for inflammatory problems of the digestive system – gastritis, peptic ulcers, regional ileitis and colitis, all of which can benefit from its regular use. It is thought to cleanse the lymph nodes, and is valuable in treating underlying toxicity in many chronic conditions e.g. enlarged lymph nodes, acne. It may be used for liver and gall bladder problems including hepatitis. Marigold is mildly oestrogenic and may be used (in combination) for period pains and to regulate menstrual bleeding (menorrhagia). The infusion makes a good wash and douche in vaginitis and vaginal thrush. Marigold plays a part in many herbal prescriptions, especially in the treatment of chronic infections, e.g. of the digestive system, womb and skin.

COMBINATIONS
With Echinacea and Nettle for chronic skin conditions; urticaria; chronic infections and chronic inflammatory states
With Wild Yam, Agnus Castus and Cramp Bark for irregular and painful periods

33 | *Carduus Marianus* – MILK THISTLE, MARY THISTLE
•••••••••••••••••••••••••••••••

Family: *Compositae*

Habitat and cultivation
Native to southern Europe, Milk Thistle thrives in waste ground and uncultivated places. It is also grown as an ornamental plant. Grows readily from seed and will self seed if allowed, in sunny positions. The seeds are collected in late summer when mature.

CONSTITUENTS
Flavonolignans (0.7%) = 'silymarin': mainly silybin, also silydianin and silychristin, Bitter principle; Polyacetylenes; Volatile oil

Key actions: Protects liver, antioxidant, stimulates bile flow, stimulates breast milk production.

Pharmacology/Research

Research from 1968 onwards has focused on the flavonolignans which exert a highly protective effect on the sinusoidal cells of the liver, supporting normal liver function and protecting against hepatotoxicity. In animal experiments, liver breakdown and death resulting from the ingestion of carbon tetrachloride, or of toxins within the Death Cap mushroom (*Amanita phalloides*), is entirely prevented if silymarin is taken beforehand or within 20 minutes of the poisoning taking place. Silymarin has been successfully used in Germany to treat cases of hepatitis and liver cirrhosis, and stimulates liver cell regeneration. A double blind clinical trial using silymarin produced statistically significant results in the treatment of Hepatitis A. Other trials have indicated effectiveness for the treatment of alcohol induced liver damage. Silymarin stabilises liver (sinusoidal) cell membranes, stimulates protein synthesis and speeds up regeneration. Milk Thistle has demonstrated antioxidant action.

Cautions: no known side effects; however Milk Thistle plants absorb large quantities of nitrate fertilisers and can cause poisoning as a result, i.e. it should be cultivated organically.

Parts used: Seeds

PREPARATIONS
Decoction rarely used
Capsules preferable – take up to 5g a day
Liquid extract (1:1) – up to 10ml a day

Key indications: Liver weakness or infection – hepatitis; liver poisoning – anti-cancer drugs, alcoholism, etc; to increase breast milk production.

Indications

Milk Thistle is the main hepato-protective and -restorative remedy. There are a number of other herbs that protect liver function Globe Artichoke

(*Cynara scolymus*) but Milk Thistle is the *most* effective. It has a place in the treatment of hepatitis A (also B and C) and jaundice, and in any situation where the liver is under stress – whether from infection, alcohol, or conventional chemotherapy prescribed for, e.g. cancer. In this last instance Milk Thistle will reduce potential damage to the liver and aid recovery from side effects once the treatment is ended. Traditionally, Milk Thistle was taken to increase breast milk production, to treat liver and bile duct problems, and was eaten as a spring tonic, providing a general cleansing regime after the winter months deprived of fresh vegetables. The flowerheads can be boiled and eaten like Artichokes. It was considered an excellent remedy for melancholia (itself associated with the liver). Gerard states in his Herbal (1597): 'My opinion is that this is the best remedy that grows against all melancholy diseases'.

COMBINATIONS
With Dandelion, Echinacea, Golden Seal for hepatitis

34 | *Urtica Dioica* – NETTLE

Family: *Urticaceae*

Habitat and cultivation

Too well known to need an introduction, Nettle barely needs to be cultivated! In the UK it is one of the commonest of all plants, being found in waste places, around the edges of fields, hedgerows and roadsides. Pick the young shoots in spring as a tonic and a vegetable, the old leaves and stems from June to August when in flower for medicinal use. The root is harvested in the autumn.

CONSTITUENTS
Herb: Flavonoids – quercitin
Amines – histamine, choline, acetylcholine, serotonin
Glucoquinone
Minerals – iron, magnesium, potassium, calcium, silicic acid
Vitamin A (beta-carotene) and C
Root: Sterols – especially stigmast-4-en-3-one

Key actions: Diuretic, tonic, astringent, antihaemorrhagic, increases breast milk production (leaf), reduces prostate enlargement (root).

Pharmacology/Research
The leaves are very nutritious containing appreciable quantities of iron, and other minerals and can be of value in anaemia. The leaves stimulate the removal of uric acid by the kidneys, thus making it useful in gout and other arthritic conditions. It is markedly diuretic, possibly due to the flavonoids and high potassium content. The glucoquinone reduces blood sugar levels and Nettle can provide adjunctive treatment in non-insulin dependent diabetes. The herb is also strongly haemostatic. Research into Nettle root has focused on its role in the treatment of enlarged prostate, the sterols being chiefly responsible for the roots activity for this condition.

Other species: The Small Nettle (*Urtica urens*) is often used inter-changeably with the ordinary Nettle, it is this Nettle which is employed in homeopathy. The Roman Nettle (*U. pilulifera*) was the species most used by the Romans for 'urtication'.

Cautions: Rare allergic reactions; no known contraindications.

Parts used: Aerial parts, root.

PREPARATIONS
Infusion (leaf) – up to 15g a day
Capsule – up to 5g a day
Tincture – up to 150ml per week
Juice – up to 30ml a day

Key indications: Gout, osteoarthritis, nosebleeds, heavy menstrual bleeding, allergies, skin problems, enlarged prostate.

Indications
Nettle is first and foremost a detoxifying herb, increasing urine output and the elimination of waste products, especially urates. It is therefore valuable in arthritic problems such as gout and osteoarthritis, especially where poor kidney function and fluid retention are a feature. In view of its significant silica content, which is readily bioavailable, Nettle will also aid connective tissue repair and regeneration. As an effective haemostatic Nettle will slow or stop bleeding and is particularly helpful for heavy menstrual bleeding. Given its high iron content this makes Nettle a key herb for chronic blood loss and the anaemia which goes with it. Nettle also has an anti-allergenic activity, and may be taken for hay fever and asthma, as well as nettle rash (urticaria)! It is often used for hay fever (with Elderflower) and finds a place in many prescriptions for skin conditions such as acne, eczema, and psoriasis. The herb is thought to improve breast milk production. The root is now a specific for enlarged prostate (often combined with Saw Palmetto). Topically, the herb can be applied to itchy skin condition, and the juice is used to treat *Nettle* stings! Dioscorides (1st century AD) lists many uses for Nettle, including the chopped leaves as a plaster for septic wounds and dog bites, the juice for nose bleeds. Over and above all this Nettle has undoubted tonic qualities and makes a nourishing and tasty vegetable similar in taste to Spinach.

COMBINATIONS
With Saw Palmetto for enlarged prostate
With Elderflower for hay fever
With Celery and Devil's Claw for gout
With Burdock, Dandelion and Echinacea for acne and other skin conditions

35 | *Alchemilla Arvensis* – PARSLEY PIERT
•••••••••••••••••••••••••••••••••••••

Family: *Rosaceae*

Habitat and cultivation
Native to Europe and North Africa, Parsley Piert grows in dry sites, including the tops of walls. The aerial parts are harvested when the plant is in flower.

CONSTITUENTS
More or less unknown
Tannins

Key actions: Diuretic, antilithic (prevention of kidney stone formation), demulcent.

Pharmacology/Research
Almost no scientific research has been undertaken into this herb.

Cautions: None known.

Parts used: Herb

PREPARATIONS
Infusion – up to 10g a day
Capsule – up to 5g a day
Tincture (1:5) 45% – up to 20ml a day

Key indications: Kidney stones, kidney weakness, chronic kidney disease, urinary tract infections, fluid retention.

Indications
Though poorly researched, and an undervalued herb, Parsley Piert is often used in British herbal medicine to treat kidney and bladder problems, especially kidney stones, and gravel where formed stones have

collected in the bladder, cause irritation and obstruct urine flow. It is questionable how much the herb can actually help to dissolve existing kidney stones (especially large ones) but it is likely that its antilithic activity is of value in the prevention of further stone formation. Being demulcent and mildly astringent it is a useful remedy for cystitis and in those prone to recurrent urinary tract infections (generally in combination with herbs such as Cornsilk or Buchu). It is probably best taken as an infusion.

COMBINATIONS
With Cornsilk for kidney stones
With Cornsilk, Buchu and Saw Palmetto for cystitis

36 | *Passiflora Incarnata* – PASSIFLORA, PASSION FLOWER
●●●●●●●●●●●●●●●●●●●●●●●●●●●●●●●●●●

Family: *Passifloraceae*

Habitat and cultivation
Native to southern parts of the USA, and central and south America, Passiflora is now extensively cultivated in Europe, notably Italy, as well as America. Related species are common garden climbers. The herb is gathered when flowering or in fruit.

CONSTITUENTS
Flavonoids (1%) – isovitexin
Chlorogenic acid
Maltol
Cyanogenic glycosides (0.01%) – gynocardin
Indole alkaloids – harman (doubtful)

80

Actions: Sedative, antispasmodic, tranquillising.

Pharmacology/Research
Though Passiflora has been fairly well researched its mode of action is poorly understood. The whole herb has established sedative, tranquillising and sleep inducing properties but the constituents responsible for these actions have not been identified. It is thought to have a GABA-like tranquillising activity within the central nervous system. The presence of the indole alkaloids is disputed, and they are not found in commercial samples.

Other species: There are approximately 400 species of *Passiflora*, the vast majority being native to the Americas. Many produce a pleasant tasting edible fruit, some have a similar sedative activity to Passion Flower. *P. quadrangularis* contains serotonin.

Cautions: Safe at normal dosage; large doses can produce drowsiness.

Parts used: Herb – leaves and flowers.

PREPARATIONS
Infusion – up to 5g a day
Capsule – up to 2.5g a day
Tincture (1:8) 45% – up to 75ml per week

Key indications: Insomnia, nervous irritability, anxiety, headache, pain.

Indications
Though the exact nature of Passiflora's action on the central nervous system is not understood it is a valuable medicine for anxiety, tension, irritability and sleeplessness, in other words for times when life has become 'too much'. Its gentle sedative activity soothes and relaxes, countering nervous overactivity and panic, and makes it a mild and non-addictive herbal tranquilliser (comparable in some ways to Valerian) useful in all states of nervous irritability or over- excitability. It may be also be

prescribed for convulsions and petit mal. As a mild analgesic it may be used to help relieve neuralgic pain such as toothache and headaches. In view of its antispasmodic action it finds use in conditions as diverse as asthma, palpitations, hypertension, period pains and muscle spasticity. Passiflora remains best known as a remedy for insomnia and disturbed sleep patterns, and is well worth trying for short-term bouts of sleeplessness.

COMBINATIONS
With Valerian for insomnia and excessive nervous excitability
With Feverfew for migraine and headache
With Chamomile for irritable bowel syndrome

37 | *Mentha X Piperita* – PEPPERMINT

Family: *Labiatae*

Habitat and cultivation
Peppermint thrives in moist situations but prefers a warm climate. Widely cultivated across the world, it is cultivated mainly for its essential oil. The herb is gathered in dry sunny weather just before flowering being quickly dried or distilled.

CONSTITUENTS
Volatile oil up to 1.5%, chiefly menthol (35-55%), menthone (10-40%)
Flavonoids – luteolin, menthoside
Phenolic acids; Triterpenes

Key actions: Carminative, spasmolytic, diaphoretic, choleretic.

Pharmacology/Research

Peppermint's medicinal activity is largely due to its volatile oil which is strongly carminative and anti-spasmodic, and has significant anti-bacterial activity. Menthol, which is antiseptic and antifungal, is the constituent chiefly responsible for the cooling and anaesthetic effect of Peppermint when applied to the skin. Paradoxically, menthone is also irritant, drawing blood flow to the skin, and therefore increasing heat where applied. The whole plant is significantly antispasmodic on the digestive system, and relaxes the stomach so allowing the passage of trapped wind upwards – i.e. burping! Detailed clinical trials have confirmed its value in the treatment of irritable bowel – mainly due to the volatile oil's spasmolytic action.

Other species: Peppermint is a mystery plant! A hybrid of Watermint (*M. aquatica*), and Spearmint (*M. spicata*), both of which have similar though milder therapeutic properties, it is not known when Peppermint was first cultivated. Menthol used as a flavouring in foods, is generally extracted from Japanese Mint (*M. arvensis var. piperescans*) which contains up to 75% menthol. There are two varieties of Peppermint – Black or English Peppermint, and a less hardy variety – White Peppermint.

Cautions: The herb has no known side effects. Not suitable for children under the age of 4.

Parts used: Herb or leaves

PREPARATIONS
Infusion – up to 10g a day (in 3-4 doses/cups)
Tincture – up to 10ml a day
Capsule: herb – up to 3g a day
Essential oil – diluted at 2% for its anaesthetic qualities on the skin

Key indications: Flatulence, bloating, irritable bowel, headaches, gastric 'flu, digestive.

Indications

Peppermint is a key herb for digestive problems, increasing the flow of digestive juices and bile, and relaxing the muscles of the gut. It has a well known ability to reduce bloating, wind, colic and griping, and to help settle and soothe an irritated bowel. In soothing the lining and the muscles of the small and large intestines it helps to ease diarrhoea, and relieve a spastic colon, which can often be the cause of constipation. Peppermint tea is a valuable remedy for sufferers of gassy, flatulent digestions, and of irritable bowel syndrome, and should be seen as a mainstay in the treatment of these conditions. It can also be used successfully where headaches or even migraines are linked to digestive weakness, perhaps combined with Rosemary or Lemon Balm.

Applied directly to the skin Peppermint and its oil has a cooling anaesthetic activity, helping to relieve pain and reduce skin sensitivity. The oil is used as an inhalant and chest rub (normally in combination e.g. with Eucalyptic oil) for respiratory infections. Though Peppermint's origin is a mystery, it has been in existence for a very long time – dried Peppermint leaves have been found in Egyptian pyramid tombs dating from around 1000BC. It was grown extensively in England in the past, Mitcham (in Surrey) mint being considered the finest.

COMBINATIONS
With Lemon Balm to aid sleep, especially when disturbed by digestive discomfort
With Elderflower for colds and 'flu
With Chamomile for spasmodic problems affecting the gastro-intestinal tract

38 | *Rubus Ideaus* – RASPBERRY LEAF

Family: *Rosaceae*

Habitat and cultivation
Native to much of Europe Raspberry grows wild in hedgerows and woodland clearings. It is much cultivated for its fruit, as far north as Norway, and is propagated by suckers.

CONSTITUENTS
Tannins
Polypeptides
Flavonoids

Actions: Astringent, aids preparation for childbirth.

Pharmacology/Research
Research conducted in the 50's onwards indicates that Raspberry leaf has a direct action on the muscles of the womb during pregnancy. Its value in preparing the womb for labour is not established but there is a great deal of anecdotal evidence to support its traditional use as a parturient. As with all tannin-rich remedies it has a marked astringent activity. It contains appreciable levels of calcium.

Cautions: In pregnancy, take only during the last three months.

Parts used: Leaves.

PREPARATIONS
Infusion – up to 15g a day
Capsule – up to 3g a day
Tincture (1:5) – up to 100ml per week

Key indications: To aid childbirth; painful or heavy menstrual bleeding; stimulates breast milk production; sore throats (as a gargle); vaginal discharge (as a douche), conjunctivitis (as an eyewash).

Indications

Raspberry leaf has traditionally been used as a remedy for the latter stages of pregnancy, being taken for roughly the last trimester at a moderate dosage (infusion – about 1 cup a day). It is thought to stimulate the longitudinal muscles of the womb and to relax the cervix, thereby increasing the effectiveness of contractions. It may also be used to relieve nausea during pregnancy and to prevent miscarriage (usually with other herbs). Its astringency makes it a valuable remedy for heavy menstrual bleeding, and it can help to reduce spasmodic period pains.

Used as an astringent wash for wounds in the past, Mrs Grieves recommends a mixture of Raspberry leaf infusion and Slippery Elm powder to speed healing of wounds, burns and irritated skin. As an infusion it may be used to relieve diarrhoea, tightening the bowel and reducing irritability e.g. in diverticulitis. Whether as a gargle, douche or eyewash it will serve well in relieving sore throats, mouth ulcers, gingivitis, vaginal discharge and conjunctivitis. It has a reputation as an oestrogenic herb and has been prescribed by herbalists for menopausal problems. Given its high calcium content it has been recommended as a long term supplement to prevent the onset of osteoporosis.

COMBINATIONS

With Black Cohosh and/or Wild Yam for spasmodic period pains
With Black Cohosh and Sage for menopausal problems
With Cranesbill for diarrhoea

39 | *Rosemary Officinalis* – ROSEMARY
•••••••••••••••••••••••••••••••••

Family: *Labiatae*

Habitat and cultivation
A native of Mediterranean Europe, Rosemary prefers a warm moderately dry climate and a sheltered site. Its name comes from the Latin *ros marinus* = sea dew. It grows throughout much of southern Europe, being cultivated as a garden and culinary plant around the world. The branches are gathered after flowering during the summer and dried in the shade.

CONSTITUENTS
Volatile oil – 1–2% (composition variable) – borneol, camphene, camphor, cineole
Flavonoids – apigenin, diosmin
Tannins: Rosmarinic acid; Diterpenes; Rosmaricine

Actions: Tonic, astringent, nervine, anti-inflammatory, carminative.

Pharmacology/Research
Rosemary's anti-inflammatory effect is due largely to rosmarinic acid and the flavonoids present; which also exert a strengthening effect on the capillaries. The herb is strongly anti-oxidant, research showing that it is particularly effective at preventing the rancidification of oils – underlining its use in cooking where it will help to prevent the decay of oils in food. Rosmaricine is a stimulant and mildly analgesic, and the whole herb has bitter and astringent properties. The volatile oil, which varies from plant to plant, is stimulant and analgesic especially when applied to the skin.

Cautions: The herb has no known side effects; the oil should be used diluted on the skin.

Parts used: Leaves.

PREPARATIONS
Infusion – up to 10g a day
Capsules – up to 3g a day
Tincture (1:5) 45% – up to 15ml a day
Lotion – the strained infusion can be used as a hair rinse, or added for an invigorating bath

Key indications: Headaches, migraine; hair growth stimulant; recovery from chronic illness; digestive weakness; lowered vitality and mild depression.

Indications
Rosemary has a central place in European herbal medicine being a warming and tonic herb, strengthening the digestion and stimulating the circulation, especially to the head. It is thought to improve memory and concentration, and has been used by students taking exams from the time of classical Greece onwards, where it was seen as the herb of Memory. Rosemary will help to relieve headaches and migraines and, by improving blood flow to the scalp, encourages hair growth. It is a valuable remedy in cases of fainting and weakness associated with deficient circulation, and can be of help in epilepsy and vertigo.

Rosemary supports recovery after long-term stress and chronic illness, and is considered a specific for debilitated states, especially if weakness and debility is also accompanied by poor circulation and digestion. It is thought to have a tonic activity on the adrenal glands. Given the stressful nature of modern life Rosemary is often prescribed for people who, though not actually ill, are 'failing to thrive'. It has always been valued as a herb to raise the spirits, and to promote a more optimistic view of life, and is certainly to be considered in cases of mild to moderate depression.

Applied externally, as a lotion or diluted essential oil, it makes a good rub for aching and rheumatic muscles; the infusion or 5 drops of the oil can be added to water for a revivifying bath; and the strained infusion can be applied and rubbed in to the scalp to encourage normal hair growth.

COMBINATIONS
With St John's Wort and Lemon Balm for depression
With Vervain and Yarrow for 'failure to thrive'
With Echinacea and Liquorice for chronic infections

40 | *Salvis Officinalis* – SAGE
•••••••••••••••••••••••

Family: *Labiatae*

Habitat and cultivation
Sage, originally from the Mediterranean region is one of those plants that is cultivated literally around the world, thriving in chalky soils and a sunny climate. The leaves should be gathered from plants up to 3-4 years old. They can be picked throughout the summer from May to August.

CONSTITUENTS
Volatile oil about 1.25% – thujone 35-60%, other monoterpenes e.g. cineole
Small quantity of sesquiterpenes
Diterpene bitters e.g. carnosol
Flavonoids
Phenolic acids and tannins

Actions: Astringent, antiseptic, aromatic, reduces sweating, digestive tonic.

Pharmacology/Research
Thujone, present in high quantities in the volatile oil of *S. officinalis* var. minor and major only, is strongly antiseptic and carminative. In excess it is highly neurotoxic. The volatile oil as a whole is anti-microbial, and reduces mucus production and muscle spasm. Sage's oestrogenic action – it relieves menopausal hot flushing and reduces breast milk production, is well documented, but the constituents responsible for these actions have not been identified. Research into Sage suggests that it has significant tranquillising activity.

Cautions: Contraindicated during pregnancy. Do not exceed recommended dosage.

Parts used: Leaves – fresh or dried.

PREPARATIONS
Infusion/gargle – up to 5g a day
Capsule – up to 2g a day
Tincture (1:5) – up to 60ml per week

Key indications: Sore throat, upper respiratory catarrh, excessive sweating, menopausal flushing and tiredness, to aid weaning and for breast engorgement, digestive tonic, diarrhoea.

Indications

Sage is seen first and foremost as a remedy for the throat, its combination of antiseptic, relaxing and astringent actions making it ideal for almost all types of sore throat. For greater effect add a pinch of Cayenne pepper (*Capsicum frutescens*). Nevertheless, Sage has a far wider range of applications than this. It is a digestive tonic and stimulant – a yin tonic in Chinese terms, making it of value in dyspepsia, diarrhoea and irritable bowel. It has a long reputation as a nerve tonic calming and stimulating the nervous system; and is a valuable remedy for irregular and scanty periods, encouraging a better flow of menstrual blood. Though Sage's hormonal action is not properly understood, there is no doubt that it has the ability to reduce sweating, and given its generally tonic and oestrogenic nature, it is an excellent remedy for the menopause – not only reducing hot flushing, but helping the body to adapt to the hormonal changes involved. Sage has been used in asthma, and the dried leaves are often included in herbal smoking mixtures for asthma. Recent *in vitro* research by Perry in Newcastle has shown that Sage and Sage oil inhibit the enzyme acetylcholinesterase (AChE) that breaks down acetylcholine. This neurotransmitter becomes deficient in the brain in Alzheimer's disease, suggesting Sage's potential as a treatment in this condition. It is unclear at present whether this activity occurs when Sage is taken orally and clinical trials are planned. All in all, its current range of uses merits the ancient saying from the mediaeval medical school at Salerno: *Salvia salvatrix* (= Sage the saviour), as well as the Spanish saying – 'Why should a man die while Sage grows in his garden?'

COMBINATIONS
With Agnus castus for menopausal problems
With Echinacea for chronic sore throat

41 | *Serenoa Serrulata* – SAW PALMETTO
••••••••••••••••••••••••••••••••

Family: *Palmaceae*

Habitat and cultivation
A small shrubby palm native to southern USA found in sand dunes and along the Atlantic and Caribbean coastline from South Carolina to Texas. The drupe is collected when ripe and dried.

CONSTITUENTS
Essential oil – 1-2%
Fixed oil
Sterols – beta-sitosterol
Flavonoids
Polysaccharides

Actions: Anti-inflammatory, tonic, endocrine agent, spasmolytic, diuretic, sedative.

Pharmacology/Research
Though a significant body of research into the activity of Saw Palmetto extract exists there is no clear understanding of how the herb works in the treatment of enlarged prostate. Saw Palmetto does not appear to have a marked effect on the enzyme (5-alpha-reductase) responsible for transforming testosterone into the more concentrated dihyrotestosterone – one of the hormones implicated in the development of enlarged prostate. The herb appears to inhibit to some extent both androgens and oestrogens – contrary to traditional views that the herb has a testosterogenic-type action

A range of clinical trials over the past 15 years have indicated that the fat-soluble extract of Saw Palmetto has a positive action in enlarged prostate, improving urine flow, bladder emptying and the need to wake at night to pass urine. Saw Palmetto has been shown in a number of clinical trials to be as effective as conventional treatment with a lower incidence of side effects. Along with Nettle root, Saw Palmetto is the preferred treatment for enlarged prostate across much of Europe.

Other species: The Maya used the roots or leaves of *S. japa*, another small palm, as a remedy for dysentery and abdominal pain. The crushed roots of *S. adamsonii* were used by Houma Indians as an eye lotion.

Cautions: Gastro-intestinal complaints can occur.

Parts used: Fruit

PREPARATIONS
Infusion – up to 3g a day
Capsule – up to 1.5g a day
Tincture (1:5) – up to 40ml per week

Key indications: Enlarged and inflamed prostate, impotence and male sterility, irritable bladder.

Indications
Traditionally, Saw Palmetto is seen as a tonic and building herb, being considered one of the few western remedies with a directly anabolic (weight building) activity. It is therefore given in cases of testicular wasting, for general debility and failure to thrive, and for other hormonal disorders. It has been seen mainly as a men's herb in the past though it may well be a useful tonic for women too. It has been called the 'plant catheter' in view of its apparent ability to tone up and strengthen the neck of the bladder, and reduce obstruction of the bladder by an enlarged prostate gland.

Though it may help in the voiding of urinary stones and 'gravel' it is used chiefly as a tonic diuretic, improving urine flow; to reverse prostate enlargement; and as a urinary antiseptic in cystitis. The herb's anti-inflammatory and anti-spasmodic activity could make it of value in the treatment of irritable bladder conditions. Saw Palmetto fruits are eaten as food by animals (and occasionally humans), and it is said that southern settlers seeing their animals grow 'sleek and fat' on the fruits, tried them out and attributed medicinal properties to it. Certainly, the fruit pulp was used as a tonic in the USA from the 19th century onwards, helping especially in debility and weakness, and as a urinary remedy, reducing prostate enlargement and relieving cystitis. It has a slightly hot, soapy and sweet taste.

COMBINATIONS
With Nettle root for benign prostate enlargement
With Echinacea and Willow for prostatitis
With Buchu and Kava Kava for irritable bladder

42 | *Hypericum Perforatum* – ST JOHN'S WORT *Y Fendigedig* (Welsh: The Blessed)
● ●

Family: *Hypericaceae*

Habitat and cultivation
Native to Britain and Europe, now naturalised throughout much of the
world, St John's Wort grows in sunny situations – meadows, roadsides and
banks, preferring a chalky soil. A perennial, it may easily be grown from
seed.

CONSTITUENTS
Dianthrone derivatives – hypericin, pseudohypericin
Flavonoids
Hyperforin
Xanthones
Oligomeric procyanidins
Coumarins
Phenolic acids – caffeic acid, chlorogenic acid
Tannins (condensed)

Actions: Anti-depressant, anti-viral, anti-inflammatory, vulnerary,
antispasmodic, cholagogue, astringent.

Pharmacology/Research

From the mid 1980's onwards there has been extensive research undertaken in to the potential value of Hypericum as a medicine. The two areas on which research has focused have been the plants antidepressant and anti-viral activity. Over 14 clinical trials, conducted between 1984 and 1993 in Germany or Austria, concluded that St John's Wort is an effective anti-depressant. In comparison with established anti-depressants the authors noted no significant difference between the two groups. The *British Medical Journal* (8.8.96) in its editorial was forced to admit that evidence for St John's Wort's activity as an anti-depressant was fairly compelling. In a clinical study against placebo in Austria, 67% of patients with mild to moderate depression improved when given an extract of St John's Wort. The authors concluded that 'due to its moderate side effects which compared to synthetic antidepressants are of minor significance only, the Hypericum extract LI 160 can be recommended for the treatment of mild to moderate depression' (Harrer and Sommer, Phytomedicine (1994) I.1). Following the experience of medical herbalists St John's Wort is also thought to have an anxiolytic effect, and short term trials have indicated its potential in anxiety states, especially when associated with depressive states. St John's Wort's anti-viral activity has been investigated largely because of its potential in treating HIV infection. Attention has focused on hypericin, which appears to have a specific activity against enveloped viruses, its strength of action being enhanced by light. In vitro studies suggest that hypericin and pseudohypericin 'interfere with assembly or processing of intact virions from infected cells . . . and directly inactivate retroviruses' (Lavie). In vivo studies indicate that hypericin and pseudohypericin are as, or more, effective than AZT and produce significantly fewer side effects. The limited clinical research into the use of St John's Wort (or hypericin-standardised extracts) suggests that the herb is worth investigating further for the treatment of HIV. A paper presented at the 1993 International Conference on AIDS (Steinbeck-Klose and Wernet) reported the findings of a trial involving 16 HIV patients at varying stages of the disease, who had taken St John's Wort for 40 months (as the sole form of treatment). During this time only 2 suffered opportunistic infection, the other 14 remained clinically stable. Over and above these areas of potential therapeutic use, St John's Wort appears to have a reasonably broad spectrum anti-bacterial action; to have an anti-inflammatory activity – one study found 'no statistical difference between the anti-inflammatory activity of Hypericum and hydrocortisone'; to stimulate wound healing; and possibly to have an anti-cancer action. Quite a herb!

Cautions: St John's Wort appears to have a low incidence of side effects. However, grazing animals have been observed to suffer from photosensitization after consuming the herb and one case of photosensitization of a woman on long term high dosage St John's Wort treatment has been reported.

Parts used: Flowering tops – picked when the flowers are opening

PREPARATIONS
Infusion/capsule – up to 4g a day
Fluid Extract (1:1) – up to 20ml per week

Key indications: Mild to moderate depression; nervous exhaustion; sciatica; shingles and post-herpetic neuralgia; viral infections.

Indications
St John's Wort is now the drug of choice in German medical practice for mild to moderate depression. In the UK it is used extensively for a range of nervous problems including anxiety, tension, depression, insomnia, and as a nerve 'restorative' – particularly for the treatment of herpes zoster. A specific for menopausal problems, treating the debility that is often an underlying factor alongside hormonal changes, and St John's Wort is also thought to be valuable for liver and gall bladder problems (more the French tradition). It may also be used in the treatment of rheumatic and arthritic conditions (anti-inflammatory action). As an anti-viral it can be used for herpetic infections, measles, hepatitis B, influenza, some colds, and HIV/AIDS. The red fixed oil makes an excellent antiseptic wound and burn healer and may be used to relieve neuralgic pain e.g. sciatica, herpes sores. The oil is also prescribed internally for gastric inflammation and peptic ulcers, and as a retention

enema in proctitis. Flowering at the time of St. John's Eve (24th June), St John's Wort has been considered a powerful medicinal herb for several thousand years. St John's Wort was known in the ancient world and valued as a vulnerary (Disocorides 1st century AD). In the Middle Ages it was known as *Fuga Daemonum*, lit. drives away demons, 'from its imagined medicinal powers in dispelling melancholy and mental illusions'. 'In the world there is not a better' treatment for deep wounds says Gerard in his Herball (1597) in which he gives a detailed prescription for preparing an oil made from the leaves, flowers and seeds. Culpepper (1652) recommends its use for wound healing, as well as the seed for 'Sciatica, the Falling-Sickness and the Palsie'. In the 19th century it fell into disrepute as a medicinal plant, though it continued to be used by herbalists in the Anglo- American tradition as a 'sedative nervine', for conditions such as sciatica, neurasthenia and depression.

COMBINATIONS
With Black Cohosh for menopausal problems including hot flushing
With Damiana for depression linked to nervous exhaustion
With Echinacea and Ginger for viral infections, especially herpes infection

43 | *Ulmus Rubra* – SLIPPERY ELM
•••••••••••••••••••••••••••

Family: *Ulmaceae*

Habitat and cultivation
A native of the northern United States and Canada, and most commonly found in the Allegheny Mountains. Slippery Elm thrives in open situations on high ground. The inner bark of the bole and branches is collected in the spring.

CONSTITUENTS
Large amounts of mucilage; starch, tannins.

Actions: Demulcent, emollient, nutrient, laxative, cough remedy.

Pharmacology/Research
There is limited research into Slippery Elm though its action as a herb containing large quantities of mucilage is well understood – at least in so far as the herb comes into direct contact with inflamed surfaces such as the skin or intestinal membranes. In this situation the effect of the herb is to soothe and 'coat' the irritated tissue, protecting it from further injury and drawing out toxins or irritants. It is thought that its effect on other mucus membranes e.g. of the urinary system, is likely to be due to a *reflex* stimulation of nerve endings in the stomach and intestines, which leads to mucus secretion in other areas of the body at the same spinal level.

Other species: Another American species, the White Elm (*Ulmus americana*) is used in a similar way to Slippery Elm, and was taken for coughs and colds by the Mohicans. The dried bark of Elm (*Ulmus spp*) has been used in Europe as a demulcent and astringent.

Cautions: None.

Parts used: Inner bark – normally available only as a powder.

PREPARATIONS
Decoction (powder): soak in hot water, about 1 heaped tsp to ½–1pt
Capsules – take with plenty of water
Poultice – often mixed with Echinacea tincture

Key indications: Gastritis and acid indigestion, hiatus hernia, peptic ulceration, diarrhoea, constipation, colitis and irritable bowel, convalescence, bronchitis and pleurisy, cystitis, as a baby food, and topically as a 'drawing' poultice.

Indications
An excellent nutrient and demulcent Slippery Elm soothes and relieves

problems as diverse as hyperacidity, gastro- enteritis, diarrhoea, bronchitis and painful cough. It may be taken regularly as a gruel in convalescence and in debilitated states, especially where the digestion is weak or overly sensitive e.g. recovery from enteric infection. It makes a good baby food. Within the gut it soothes inflammation, and colic/spasm, and will help in almost all problems affecting the colon – constipation, diverticulitis, irritable bowel an ulcerative colitis as well as painful (internal) haemorrhoids. May be prescribed for all chest conditions from simple coughs and bronchitis to pleurisy and tuberculosis – wherever a demulcent action is required. A demulcent to consider in urinary problems such as chronic cystitis. Topically, Slippery Elm is emollient and protective, and makes a very effective 'drawing' poultice – for deep splinters, whitlows, boils, and the like – often mixed with Echinacea or Marigold tincture.

COMBINATIONS
With Thyme for chronic coughs
With Cranesbill for diarrhoea
With Chamomile for gastritis and peptic ulceration

44 | *Thymus Vulgaris –* THYME, GARDEN THYME
•••••••••••••••••••••••••••

Family: *Labiatae*

Habitat and cultivation
Thyme is an 'improved' variety of Wild Thyme native to countries bordering the Mediterranean. It is cultivated extensively as a kitchen herb and for its essential oil. It prefers light chalky soils and a dry situation and is harvested in the summer.

CONSTITUENTS
Volatile oil, with variable content – thymol, carvacrol, cineole, bomeol
Flavonoids – apigenin, luteolin
Tannin

Actions: Antiseptic, tonic, spasmolytic, expectorant, worm repellant.

Pharmacology/Research
The volatile oil is strongly antiseptic, thymol in particular being an effective antifungal agent. It is also an expectorant and expels worms. Thymol, carvacrol and the flavonoids are spasmolytic. Recent research in Scotland suggests that Thyme and its volatile oil are markedly tonic, supporting the body's normal function and countering the effects of aging.

Other species: There are many other Thyme species, all with a different essential oil content. Mother of Thyme (*T. serpyllum*) is often used interchangeably with Thymus.

Cautions: The oil should *not* be taken internally.

Parts used: Leaves/Aerial Parts – an excellent tea for coughs and chest infections.

PREPARATIONS
Infusion: fresh leaves – up to 10g per day; dried leaves – up to 5g per day
Capsules – up to 2g a day
Tincture(1:5) – up to 8ml a day
Essential oil – diluted to 5% maximum as an antiseptic and for lice and scabies

Key indications: Bronchitis, cough, whooping cough, recovery from chest infection, asthma, threadworms, fungal infections.

Indications
Being such a common garden herb Thyme's qualities as a medicine tend

to be underappreciated. In fact it is a key herb for chest infections such as bronchitis, whooping cough and pleurisy, and makes an excellent tonic (and to a lesser degree immune stimulant) in chronic, especially fungal, infections. The tea is pleasant tasting, especially when flavoured with honey, and will bring relief to coughs, minor throat and chest infections. The fresh leaves can be chewed to relieve sore throats. It is commonly used with other herbs e.g. Lobelia, for asthma, particularly in children, where its invigorating, tonic qualities balance the often sedative effect of many herbal medicines used for asthma. Apply Thyme topically for arthritic and rheumatic aches and pains – the infusion or diluted essential oil (max 5%) should be massaged well into the area; also for sciatica; as an antifungal lotion for ringworm, athletes foot, thrush and other fungal infections; scabies and lice; and as a warming and stimulating bath (infusion is best). It is also a good remedy for worms, commonly being given to treat thread worms in children. In short a valuable yet undervalued remedy, for all manner of respiratory problems, as an anti-fungal and an effective tonic. Thyme has a place in all gardens and medicine chests!

COMBINATIONS
With Echinacea and Elecampane for bronchitis and other chest infections
With Lobelia for asthma

45 | *Valeriana Officinalis* – VALERIAN
••••••••••••••••••••••••••••••

Family: *Valerianaceae*

Habitat and cultivation
Native to Europe and northern Asia, Valerian thrives in damp places such as river banks. It is cultivated in central and eastern Europe, the roots being dug up in autumn.

CONSTITUENTS
Volatile oil up to 1.4%
– bornyl acetate, B-caryphyllene
– sesquiterpenes including valerenic acid, valerenal, valeranone
Valepotriates (iridoids) – valtrate, isovaltrate
Alkaloids

Actions: Sedative, relaxant, spasmolytic, anxiolytic, hypotensive.

Pharmacology/research
Valerian is an acknowledged sedative and relaxant, though the constituents responsible for this action have not been identified. At first the valepotriates were considered the main active constituents but their presence is not necessary for the plant's sedative activity; the same is true to a lesser degree for the sesquiterpenes which are markedly sedative (valerenic acid especially) and antispasmodic. The main active constituents responsible for the anxyiolytic activity are yet to be identified. Animal and human studies indicate that Valerian's sleep inducing action has a beneficial effect on both length and quality of sleep, reducing the time it takes to get off to sleep and frequency of wakening. The root is sedative and is thought not to impair driving or use of machinery, or usually to produce drowsiness as a side effect. In other words, its anxiolytic action is mild and bears no comparison with benzodiazapenes such as Valium. It is therefore a very useful remedy for anxiety, stress-related disorders and over-excitability. It neither interferes with normal function, nor leads to addiction. It has an established action in lowering blood pressure. For a very useful summary see Corrigan D., *Sleep and Relaxation*, Amberwood (1996).

Cautions: Can cause drowsiness. As a side note, a 1994 report by the National Poisons Unit (Medical Toxicology Unit at Guy's Hospital, London) included details of 24 people who had attempted suicide using herbal sleeping tablets – all of which are likely to have contained Valerian as a major ingredient. The only side effect reported was drowsiness!

Parts used: Root and rhizome.

PREPARATIONS
Decoction – up to 4g a day
Capsule – up to 2g a day
Tincture (1:5) – up to 100ml per week

Key indications: Stress, anxiety, nervous tension, panic attacks, overexcitability, insomnia, muscular tension, high blood pressure, asthma, irritable bowel, period pains.

Indications
High stress levels seem to be endemic to late 20th century living and Valerian therefore has an increasingly frequent role to play in herbal practice. Thought of as the 'herbal tranquilliser', its ability to reduce nervous excitability and overactivity – especially when the patient cannot 'switch off' is of great value, especially in chronic 'worriers' and perfectionists. It calms the mind, rather than sedating the body, and has a huge range of applications. It will relax over contracted tissues – so helping in musculo-skeletal problems such as frozen shoulder, back pain and neck tension, as well as asthma, colic, irritable bowel, period pains and so on; it will relieve symptoms of anxiety such as tremor, panic, palpitations and sweating; and makes a useful remedy in insomnia whether due to anxiety or overexcitement. Valerian is also a specific for high blood pressure caused by stress and anxiety, though it is always combined with other herbs for this condition. In short, any situation caused by nervous overactivity can benefit from Valerian.

Opinion differs amongst medical herbalists about the appropriate dosage level for Valerian. While large doses may be reasonable for some robust people, even 5g per week may be too much for more delicate 'nervous' constitutions and have a potentially depressive activity (its use is not normally advisable in depression).

Perhaps this difference reflects a misunderstanding of Valerian's proper application – it is most useful in larger doses for strong, overactive individuals who will not be suppressed by its sedative edge. In nervously (or adrenally) exhausted individuals more than a small dosage may impair mood. My own personal observation is that many patients suffering from long-term anxiety are also suffering to a limited degree from depression (presumably as a result of neuro-endocrine exhaustion). In this situation Valerian needs to be combined with tonic herbs such as Rosemary, Oats or St John's Wort. Lastly, if taking Valerian for the first time it is generally wise to start at a low dosage and work up.

COMBINATIONS
With Hawthorn for high blood pressure linked to stress
With St John's Wort for insomnia and anxiety linked with depression
With Chamomile for digestive and menstrual cramping pains

46 | *Verbena Officinalis* – VERVAIN
••••••••••••••••••••••••••

Family: *Verbenaceae*

Habitat and cultivation
Vervain grows through much of Europe, preferring a chalky soil and sunny position. It is easily cultivated in temperate climates.

CONSTITUENTS
Bitter iridoids – verbenin, verbenalin
Essential oil
Alkaloids; Mucilage; Tannin

Key actions: Nervine, tonic, spasmolytic, mild sedative, cholagogue, galactagogue (stimulates breast milk).

Pharmacology/Research
Poorly researched Vervain has established bitter and digestive stimulant properties, being emetic at high doses. Verbenalin is a mild purgative and oxytocic in isolation. The whole plant is thought to have a para-

sympathetic action – improving vegetative and restorative aspects of normal body function. The iridoids are cholagogic. In view of its botanical closeness to Agnus Castus (*Vitex agnus castus*) and its apparent ability to stimulate breast milk production, it is interesting to speculate whether Vervain may not also have significant hormonal activity.

Other species: A number of other *Verbena* are used medicinally, such as *V. domingensis* used in the Caribbean as a bitter tonic, for wounds and for headaches, and the north American *V. hastata*, used by surgeons in the Revolutionary Wars as an emetic and expectorant.

Cautions: Can cause vomiting if taken in excess. Avoid during pregnancy.

Parts used: Herb

PREPARATIONS
Infusion – up to 5g a day
Capsule – up to 2.5g a day
Tincture (1:5) 45% – up to 10ml a day

Key indications: Nervous tension and exhaustion, anxiety and stress, weak digestive function, headaches and migraines, menstrual problems.

Indications
Vervain is a nervine tonic and restorative, especially valuable in relieving nervous tension. It is thought to have antidepressant activity, though it is more specific for anxiety and nervous exhaustion following long term stress. At the same time it has a strongly tonic effect on the digestion, improving absorption, and therefore nourishment to the body's tissues. By strengthening the body and aiding mental and emotional relaxation, the herb is ideal for recovery from chronic illness where nervous weakness and exhaustion are a feature. It may also be given for asthma, insomnia and headaches. It is used in traditional Chinese medicine to treat migraines connected with the menstrual cycle, and is also valuable for pre-menstrual syndrome, reducing emotional irritability and distress (though it is probably best not used in severe period pains). Vervain finds

use in the treatment of fevers especially at the beginning of 'flus; during labour to encourage contractions; to increase breast milk production; for gallstones and jaundice, being thought by some authorities to be a specific for gall bladder pains; as a mild laxative; and lastly as a dentifrice, the powder being a useful ingredient for toothpastes and powders. All in all a very useful and easily undervalued remedy.

COMBINATIONS
With Rosemary and Thyme for nervous exhaustion
With Agnus castus for pre-menstrual syndrome

47 | *Dioscorea Spp* – WILD YAM ROOT
• •

Family: *Dioscoreaceae*

Habitat and cultivation
Wild Yam is a deciduous, perennial vine which climbs to a height of up to 6m. A major food plant with potato-like tubers, it is native to north and central America especially Mexico and is extensively cultivated.

CONSTITUENTS
Steroidal saponins – mainly dioscine
Phytosterols – including B-sitosterol
Alkaloids
Tannins
Starch

Actions: Anti-spasmodic, anti-inflammatory, anti-rheumatic, oestrogenic, diaphoretic, diuretic, expectorant.

Pharmacology/Research

Wild Yam is the original plant source of dioscine, a steroid-type molecule that led to the development of a number of steroid hormones and of the contraceptive pill. First identified by Japanese scientists in 1936, this discovery paved the way for the laboratory production, firstly of progesterone – one of the main female sex hormones, and then of cortico-steroid hormones such as cortisone. Wild Yam's steroidal saponins have an oestrogenic action and the herb is therefore useful in treating menstrual and menopausal problems. Contrary to much popular opinion the steroidal saponins in Wild Yam do not have a progesterogenic activity. The steroidal saponins are also anti-inflammatory, tending to confirm the use of Wild Yam for arthritic and rheumatic conditions.

Parts used: Underground parts – root and tuber.

PREPARATIONS
Decoction – up to 5g a day
Capsule – up to 2g a day
Tincture – up to 50ml per week

Key indications: Menopausal and menstrual problems such as hot flushing, pre-menstrual syndrome, spasmodic period pain and polycystic ovary syndrome; osteoarthritis; rheumatoid arthritis; irritable bowel syndrome.

Indications

Known as Colic root or Rheumatism root to American settlers, the Mayas and the Aztecs used the plant to relieve period pains and the pain of childbirth. There is no evidence that the plant was used as a contraceptive in the past but there is no question as to its value in relieving spasmodic pains such as menstrual cramps. It will also help to relieve muscle spasms and pains – whether affecting skeletal or smooth muscle – and is effective in relieving cramps affecting the intestines. Wild Yam's other main therapeutic uses are for arthritis and rheumatism, where its combination of anti- inflammatory and anti-spasmodic activity makes it a valuable remedy – reducing inflammation and relaxing stiffened and painful muscles in the affected area. It can be beneficial in treating a number of digestive problems including gallbladder inflammation, irritable bowel syndrome and diverticulitis; and it has a persistent reputation as a good tonic herb for the liver. All in all a very useful medicinal plant.

COMBINATIONS
With Devil's Claw and Willow Bark for inflammatory arthritic conditions
With Capsicum and Black Cohosh for osteoarthritis
With Agnus Castus for pre-menstrual syndrome

48 | *Salix Alba* – WILLOW BARK
• •

Family: *Salicaeae*

Habitat and cultivation
The Willow tree is found through most of Europe, North Africa and Asia, and thrives in damp and wet areas, often along river banks. The bark is stripped from 2-5 year old branches in the spring (April-May).

CONSTITUENTS
Phenolic glycosides – up to 11% – including salicin
Flavonoids; Tannins – up to 20%

Actions: Anti-inflammatory, analgesic, anti-pyretic, anti-rheumatic, astringent.

Pharmacology/Research
Research into Salix began a long time ago – salicin was first isolated from the tree in 1838. Salicin became the forerunner of aspirin (= acetylsalicylic acid), first produced as a chemical in 1899. Salicin (and

the phenolic glycosides in general) has similar analgesic and anti-inflammatory properties to aspirin – inhibiting prostaglandin production and relieving pain, reducing fevers. However, as the phenolic compounds are taken within the context of the bark as a whole (which is markedly astringent), and salicin is absorbed in the duodenum rather than the stomach, no irritation of the stomach lining occurs (a common side effect of aspirin when taken in large doses or over an extended period of time). Salicin does *not* however, have the blood thinning properties of aspirin. There has been next to no research on the bark as a whole.

Other species: Many other species of Salix are used interchangeably with White Willow e.g. Crack Willow (*S. fragilis*). In North American herbal medicine Black Willow (*S. nigra*) is used as an aphrodisiac or sexual depressant. *S. acmophylla* is used in herbal medicine in the Indian sub continent as a remedy for fevers.

Cautions: Those allergic to aspirin should avoid Willow Bark.

Parts used: Bark – from young branches.

PREPARATIONS
Decoction – up to 5g a day
Capsule – up to 2.5g a day
Tincture (1:5) – up to 100ml per week

Key indications: Pain and inflammation of arthritis, pain, excessive sweating, fever, headache.

Indications
Willow Bark is specific for rheumatic and arthritic inflammation, and for pain brought on by such inflammation (or degeneration) e.g. arthritic and rheumatic pain affecting the knees, hips and back. It may also be used for gout, ankylosing spondylitis and psoriatic arthropathy. Experience suggests that Willow Bark will not reverse arthritic problems on its own and it should always be used in combination with other herbs such as Celery seed. It is only mildly analgesic. A good fever remedy, taken in

combination with diaphoretic herbs such as Peppermint, it will aid the management and lower high fevers. It may be used symptomatically to ease headaches and head pain. Dioscorides (1st century AD) suggests taking 'Willow leaves, mashed with a little pepper and drunk with wine to relieve lower back pain'.

COMBINATIONS

With Celery seeds for osteoarthritis and joint pain

With Devil's Claw and/or Black Cohosh for rheumatoid and other inflammatory arthritis

With Feverfew for headache and migraine

49 | *Hamamelis Virginiana* – WITCH HAZEL

Family: *Hamamelidaceae*

Habitat and cultivation

Witch Hazel is a woodland tree indigenous to the north-eastern United States and Canada. It has also become a fairly common garden tree in Europe. It may be cultivated from cuttings or seed. The leaves are gathered in the summer.

CONSTITUENTS (Leaves)

Tannins (8-10%), hydrolysable and condensed, and including proanthocyanins

Flavonoids; Bitter principle; Volatile oil

Key actions: Astringent, anti–inflammatory, haemostatic (stops bleeding).

Pharmacology/Research

Witch Hazel's therapeutic activity is largely due to the presence of significant levels of tannins. The astringency produced by tannins leads to the tightening up of proteins within the skin and across the surface of cuts and abrasions, drawing the skin together and laying down a protective coating. The proanthocyanins and flavonoids have a restorative activity on the capillaries beneath the skin and increase resistance to inflammation. When distilled Witch Hazel retains its astringency suggesting that astringent agents other than tannins are present.

Cautions: Not recommended for internal use; if taken internally use for no more than 1 week at a time. Do not apply topically to wounds or to burns where the surface of the skin has been removed.

Parts used: Leaves (more astringent than the bark), bark of twigs, twigs.

PREPARATIONS
Infusion/decoction – as a lotion for topical use, e.g. varicose veins
Distilled water – best for everyday use on over-relaxed skin
Ointment – for haemorrhoids
Spray – with e.g. Ti-tree oil for inflamed and infected skin
Poultice (soak in infusion or decoction)

Key indications: Lax and inflamed skin conditions; bruises and spontaneous bruising; sprains and hernias; raised capillaries; varicose veins; haemorrhoids; sore eyes and conjunctivitis; nose bleeds.

Indications
A valuable remedy for many inflamed and tender skin conditions Witch Hazel may be used as much as a cosmetic as a medine. Apply as a lotion or poultice to skin blemishes, roughened or sagging skin, to abrasions, and to treat problems underlying the skin such as raised capillaries, sprains and swellings. Its strong astringent action relieves inflammation and tightens up lax or distended tissues, making it particularly useful for varicose veins – the lotion, and haemorrhoids – the ointment. Distilled Witch Hazel water makes an effective eyewash for tired, bruised and inflamed eyes. In traditional North American herbal medicine, Witch Hazel bark was applied as a poultice to treat tumours and inflammations (especially of the

eye), and taken internally for haemorrhage and heavy menstrual bleeding. Its use was developed by Eclectic and other herbalists in the USA in the 19th century and popularised as Pond's Cold Cream – essentially a Witch Hazel product. Witch Hazel is still recognised in many Pharmacopoeias, principally as distilled Witch Hazel water.

COMBINATIONS
With Marigold for inflamed skin
With Echinacea for weeping skin infections
Equal parts of distilled Witch Hazel and Rose waters as a skin tonic

50 | *Artemisia Absinthium* – WORMWOOD

Family: *Compositae*

Habitat and cultivation
Native to maritime regions of Europe, Wormwood is naturalised in eastern America and central Asia. A wayside plant which will only thrive in a sunny position. Propagated by dividing the roots in autumn or from seed, and cultivated in temperate regions.

CONSTITUENTS
Volatile oil – thujone (up to 70%), azulenes
Sesquiterpenes
Sesquiterpene lactones (non-volatile) including germacranolides such as costunolide, ridentin; guaianolides – (azulenes) artabsin, artabsinthin; santanolides – santonin
Flavonoids; Phenolic acids; Lignans

Key actions: Aromatic bitter, improves bile flow, antiparasitic (intestinal worms), tonic to stomach, anti-inflammatory, stimulant and mild anti-depressant.

Pharmacology/Research

Wormwood contains a 'cocktail' of active ingredients many of which are profoundly bitter, stimulating the bitter taste receptors on the tongue and reflexly leading (via the vagus nerve) to gastrin release, increased stomach and intestinal secretions and increased production of bile by the liver. The azulenes are anti-inflammatory; the sesquiterpene lactones have an anti-tumour effect, and are strongly insecticidal; thujone is toxic in large quantities being stimulant to the central nervous system in small doses but highly toxic to nerve tissue in excess. The germacranolides have an anti-tumour action. The guaianolides are insecticidal. The santanolides counter intestinal worms.

Other species: There are many medicinally useful *Artemisia* species including *A. abrotanum, A. annua, A. capillaris, A. dranunculis,* and *A. vulgaris.*

Cautions: Use in *very small* doses only, generally for no more than 2-3 months maximum at a time. Do not take during pregnancy or if peptic ulceration or significant gastritis is present. Use with caution and at low dosage only in high blood pressure and where the heart is weak. Do not take if epileptic.

Parts used: Herb

PREPARATIONS
Infusion – so unpalatable as to be undrinkable
Tincture (1:5) – recommended maximum of 10 drops before meals three times a day
Capsule – up to 100mg a day before meals
Though the taste is very bitter this is one of the few cases where actually tasting the herb rather than swallowing it, e.g. as a capsule, is preferable, as the taste itself will stimulate digestive activity.

Key indications: Weak and windy digestions; to increase stomach acid secretion especially in the second half of life when digestive 'fire' is declining; gastric and intestinal infections; gall bladder and liver disease (*not* if the gall bladder is obstructed).

Indications

Used in small doses Wormwood is a safe and extremely effective medicine for those with weak and underactive digestions. By increasing saliva and stomach acid production it aids sound digestion (thus its traditional use in Vermouths) and as a result increases the gastro-intestinal tract's ability to resist infection and parasites. This may be significant in a number of conditions such as atopic asthma and eczema, and chronic fatigue, as they are associated with impaired hydrochloric acid production and a raised stomach pH. Though contraindicated in peptic ulceration, Wormwood could be used in small doses to counter Heliobacter infection. It stimulates appetite and reduces nausea and vomiting.

Its ability to stimulate bile contributes to its ability to relieve wind, bloating and burping – the latter being associated with poor bile flow and gall bladder problems. If taken regularly as drops Wormwood slowly strengthens digestive activity and aids return to full vitality after prolonged illness. It may be taken during infections, and in combination with other herbs can help to prevent dysenteric infections. The herb has a reputation as an anti-depressant, especially where this is associated with poor liver function. Artemisia annua, a close relative, is a potent antimalarial. Wormwood itself makes a good insecticide and insect repellant – dried branches are traditionally placed in drawers to repel moths. It is a moderately effective remedy for worms – threadworms and pinworms, in children especially, though must be used with considerable caution in children.

Wormwood may be used in the short term to stimulate the onset of an absent or 'stuck' period. As with all bitters it is a useful remedy for treating feverish states. It is commonly included in prescriptions for cancer treatment. All in all an excellent example of how complex and multi-faceted a single herb may be.

COMBINATIONS
To stimulate menstruation where period is 'stuck' with Helonias and Yarrow
For gastro-intestinal infections – with Golden Seal, Echinacea and Ginger

OTHER BOOKS FROM AMBERWOOD PUBLISHING ARE:

Aromatherapy Lexicon – The Essential Reference by Geoff Lyth and Sue Charles is a colourful, fun way to learn about Aromatherapy. £4.99.

Aromatherapy – A Guide for Home Use by Christine Westwood. All you need to know about essential oils and using them. £1.99.

Aromatherapy – for Stress Management by Christine Westwood. Covering the use of essential oils for everyday stress-related problems. £3.50.

Aromatherapy – For Healthy Legs and Feet by Christine Westwood. A guide to the use of essential oils for the treatment of legs and feet. £2.99.

Aromatherapy – Simply For You by Marion Del Gaudio Mak. A clear, simple and comprehensive guide to Aromatherapy for beginners. £1.99.

Aromatherapy – The Baby Book by Marion Del Gaudio Mak. An easy to follow guide to massage for the infant or child. £3.99

Aromatherapy – A Nurses Guide by Ann Percival SRN. The ultimate, safe, lay guide to the natural benefits of Aromatherapy. Including recipes and massage techniques for many medical conditions and a quick reference chart. £2.99.

Aromatherapy – A Nurses Guide for Women by Ann Percival SRN. Concentrates on women's health for all ages. Including sections on PMT, menopause, infertility, cellulite. £2.99.

Aromatherapy – Essential Oils in Colour by Rosemary Caddy Bsc Hons, ARCS MISP is a unique book depicting the chemistry of Essential oils. £9.99.

Aroma Science – The Chemistry & Bioactivity of Essential Oils by Dr Maria Lis-Balchin. With a comprehensive list of the Oils and scientific analysis. Includes sections on the sense of smell and the history of Aromatherapy. £4.99.

Plant Medicine – A Guide for Home Use (New Edition) by Charlotte Mitchell MNIMH. A guide to home use giving an insight into the wonderful healing qualities of plants. £2.99.

Woman Medicine – Vitex Agnus Castus by Simon Mills MA, FNIMH. The story of the herb that has been used for centuries in the treatment of women's problems. £2.99.

Ancient Medicine – Ginkgo Biloba (New Edition) by Dr Desmond Corrigan BSc(Pharms), MA, Phd, FLS, FPSI. Improved memory, circulation and concentration are associated with Ginkgo and explained in this book. £2.99.

Indian Medicine – The Immune System by Dr Desmond Corrigan BSc(Pharms), MA, Phd, FLS, FPSI. An intriguing account of the history of the plant called Echinacea and its power to influence the immune system. £2.99.

Herbal Medicine for Sleep & Relaxation by Dr Desmond Corrigan BSc(Pharms), MA, PhD, FLS, FPSI. A guide to the natural sedatives as an alternative to orthodox drug therapies, drawing on the latest medical research, presented in an easy reference format. £2.99.

Herbal First Aid by Andrew Chevallier BA, MNIMH. A beautifully clear reference book of natural remedies and general first aid in the home. £2.99.

Natural Taste – Herbal Teas, A Guide for Home Use by Andrew Chevallier BA, MNIMH. Contains a comprehensive compendium of Herbal Teas gives information on how to make it, its benefits, history and folklore. £3.50.

Garlic– How Garlic Protects Your Heart by Prof E. Ernst MD, PhD. Used as a medicine for over 4500 years, this book examines the latest scientific evidence supporting Garlic's effect in reducing cardiovascular disease, the Western World's number one killer. £3.99.

Insomnia – Doctor I Can't Sleep by Dr Adrian Williams FRCP. Written by one of the world's leading sleep experts, Dr Williams explains the phenomenon of sleep and sleeping disorders and gives advice on treatment. With 25% of the adult population reporting difficulties sleeping – this book will be essential reading for many. £2.99.

Signs & Symptoms of Vitamin Deficiency by Dr Leonard Mervyn BSc, PhD, C.Chem, FRCS. A home guide for self diagnosis which explains and assesses Vitamin Therapy for the prevention of a wide variety of diseases and illnesses. £2.99.

Causes & Prevention of Vitamin Deficiency by Dr Leonard Mervyn BSc, PhD, C.Chem, FRCS. A home guide to the Vitamin content of foods and the depletion caused by cooking, storage and processing. It includes advice for those whose needs are increased due to lifestyle, illness etc. £2.99.

Eyecare Eyewear – For Better Vision by Mark Rossi Bsc, MBCO. A complete guide to eyecare and eyewear including an assessment of the types of spectacles and contact lenses available and the latest corrective surgical procedures. £3.99.

Arthritis and Rheumatism by Dr John Cosh FRCP, MD. Covers all forms of Arthritis, its affects and the treatments available. £4.95.

Notes

Notes

Notes

Notes